£1

D1078653

Burns Trauma Nursing Procedures

Chrissie Bosworth BSc (Hons) RGN
Nurse Teacher, School of Nursing and Midwifery
Faculty of Medicine and Health Science
University of Nottingham

BELONGS TO
DEWSBURY HEALTH
STAFF LIBRARY

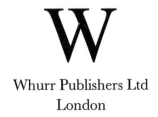

Whurr Publishers Ltd
London

© 1997 Whurr Publishers Ltd
First published 1997 by
Whurr Publishers Ltd
19B Compton Terrace, London N1 2UN, England

British Library Cataloguing in Publication Data
A catalogue record for this book is available from the
British Library.

ISBN 1 86156 009 5

Printed and bound in the UK by Athenaeum Press Ltd,
Gateshead, Tyne & Wear

Contents

Acknowledgements

The author wishes to acknowledge and express her gratitude to a number of people whose personal contributions and support have been invaluable in the production of this book.

The nursing staff from the Burns Unit at the City Hospital (NHS) Trust, Nottingham, especially Gale Harvey, Julie Ledger, Deborah Raynor, Jane Roe and Deborah Beeby (formerly senior staff nurse) for their contributions and expertise in writing these procedures.

Pip Harris, formerly Senior Nurse Clinical Development and Neville Lees, formerly Chief Nurse Advisor, from Nottingham Health Authority for their direction and encouragement in the early stages to get the project off the ground.

Clare Ashton, Director of Nursing at the City Hospital (NHS Trust), Nottingham for providing the support and resources for undertaking this project.

Members of the General Nursing Procedures Committee (City Hospital, University Hospital and Nottingham Health Care Trusts), and nursing staff from the Adult Intensive Care Units at the City Hospital and University Hospital (NHS Trusts), Nottingham, especially Susan Bowler and Pauline Hiller (formerly Sister AICU, University Hospital) for allowing me to adapt some of their original work.

A special thanks to Lizzie Stapleton from the Nursing Development Centre at the City Hospital (NHS Trust), Nottingham for her support in typing and retyping the manuscript.

Finally, to my husband Philip Bousfield for his love, faith, understanding and support throughout what has been a challenging and exciting experience.

Thank-you everyone for supporting my venture, it has been much appreciated.

Chrissie Bosworth, BSc (Hons), RGN,

Preface

Caring for individuals who have sustained burn trauma is a challenging, yet rewarding experience for nurses. In the last twenty years burn care has changed dramatically, reflecting advances in research, technology and the move towards professional status in nursing. Subsequently, the nurse involved in burn care needs to possess a combination of specialised knowledge and skills across a variety of clinical areas of nursing, namely emergency care, critical care, continuing care, infection control, nutritional care, wound care, psychological care, rehabilitation and caring for individuals requiring plastic and reconstructive surgery.

Nurses caring for individuals following burn trauma range from learners and novices with little or no experience, to expert nurses with advanced education and experience in burn care. Therefore, this book has been designed as a resource for all levels of nurses caring for individuals who have sustained a burn injury. It encompasses a variety of aspects of care and endeavours to assist nurses to base their specialist clinical practice on research based principles. It will also prove to be an additional resource for those nurses undertaking post registration diploma and degree level programmes in burns nursing, trauma and critical care.

The chosen format includes an introductory section which aims to provide a brief review of relevant literature, details a list of the equipment required for each procedure, describes step by step actions with supporting rationale using a research based approach and provides illustrations, together with a reference list and suggestions for further reading at the end of each chapter. The format will enable the user to utilise the procedures within the clinical environment relating both theory to practice whilst using a research based approach to maintain the high standards of nursing care our patients deserve.

Chrissie Bosworth BSc (Hons), RGN
Formerly Clinical Nurse Specialist, Burns Unit, City Hospital (NHS Trust),
Nottingham

Chapter 1
Advice pertaining to procedures

1. General guidelines: before, during and after the procedure

The general guidelines are applicable to a wide range of clinical procedures and are given separately to minimise repetition in later chapters. For guidance on all aspects of nursing practice refer to the Code of Professional Conduct (UKCC 1992).

Action	Rationale
Assess individual patients for factors which may affect the undertaking/outcome of the procedure. For example: – Pain – Anxiety level – Level of understanding – Physical condition – Mobility – Special procedures e.g. preoperative preparation – Potential contraindications and/or complications.	May influence choice of procedure/position patient can adopt during/following the procedure and may influence observation/nursing care required.
Give an appropriate explanation regarding the procedure in accordance with the patient's level of understanding.	Information can reduce anxiety and help a person cope with a stressful situation (Lazarus and Averill, 1972).
Obtain permission where possible prior to undertaking the procedure.	Working on the premise that to touch a person without their permission is unlawful.

Action	Rationale
N.B. It is the responsibility of the medical staff to obtain consent for procedures which they will perform.	Patients should be given relevant information where possible and understand what they are being asked to agree to, prior to commencement of the procedure (Tschudin, 1989). The importance of effective communication in nursing care is well documented (Bridge and MacLeod Clark, 1981). Advice on physical coping strategies may be appropriate (Finesilver, 1979).
Ensure privacy is maintained at all times.	Privacy is important to minimise embarrassment and preserve the patient's dignity.
For aseptic techniques prepare the environment and equipment required considering relevant ward activities.	Timing linked to activities of the ward may minimise airborne organisms in the sterile field, e.g. domestic cleaning, bed making.
Clean trolleys, wash hands and check sterile packages.	See sections 2, 3 and 4 below.
Prepare the patient for the specific procedure. Record baseline observations where relevant.	See relevant guidelines/procedures. Enables comparison with post-procedural observations and early detection of change in condition.
Position the patient appropriately and ensure the patient is comfortable. This also applies *during and after* procedure.	
Perform/assist with procedure.	See relevant guidelines/procedures, e.g. wound dressing, insertion of epidural cannula.
Monitor the patient's condition during and after procedures.	See relevant guidelines/procedures/ instructions from medical practitioner.
Clear the environment of used equipment.	See section 5 below.
Document procedure (where relevant) and modify nursing care plan appropriately.	Effective communication of information is essential for continuity and effectiveness of care.
Provide the patient with further information and ongoing support where appropriate.	Effective communication of information is essential for continuity and effectiveness of care.

2. Procedure for handwashing

Handwashing is the single most important factor in the prevention of cross infection, particularly in hospitals. Attention must be paid to the method of handwashing in order to cleanse *all* surfaces adequately. See Figure 1.1 for the areas most commonly neglected.

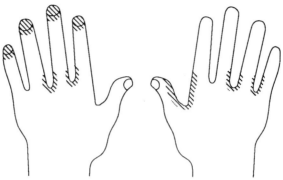

Figure 1.1 *The areas most commonly neglected in hand washing.*

Handwashing Agents	Indications For Use
Social handwash – Liquid soap.	Before and after most general duties including food handling, bedmaking, toileting.
– Alcohol hand-rub.	May be used where handwash facilities are unavailable or inadequate, or between procedures.
Hygienic handwash – Antiseptic soap.	Prior to invasive procedures, e.g. insertion of cannulae, etc.
	Prior to minor surgical procedures.
	After attending to a patient in isolation.
	In any area where more thorough antisepsis is required e.g. Burns Unit.
– Soap and water followed by alcohol hand-rub.	Where access to antiseptic soap is restricted or unavailable.
Surgical scrub – Antiseptic soap.	Prior to gowning and gloving in an ultra-clean environment, e.g. Burns Unit operating theatre.
	This is essentially a longer lasting and more thorough and extensive version of the hygienic handwash.

3. Procedure for aseptic technique

The term 'aseptic technique' is used to describe methods which have been developed to prevent contamination of susceptible sites in the operating theatre, ward environment and other treatment areas. This is achieved by ensuring that only sterile instruments and fluids make contact with these sites and that the risks of airborne contamination are also minimised.

As a general rule, any procedure which involves penetration of the skin, exposure of wounds or instrumentation should be performed using sterile materials. If there is a need to cut a sterile dressing, in order that it conforms to the wound, then sterile scissors must be used.

The single most important factor in any aseptic technique is meticulous attention to handwashing prior to the procedure, regardless of whether or not gloves are used.

Aseptic technique should always be undertaken using sterile dressings and instruments, as supplied by sterile services. Sterility is ascertained by a sterile autoclave tape, which is clear when unsterile, and produces a brown diagonal line when sterile. Packs should be clean, dry, dust proof and have an intact seal.

User's attempts to sterilise equipment should be discouraged apart from agreed specialist areas where autoclaves are regularly maintained. It is important to recognise that (with a few exceptions) immersing equipment in disinfectants will only render them disinfected *not* sterile and this procedure must *never* be adopted for use on instruments used during an aseptic technique. The sterile pack should be opened carefully using either forceps supplied or with washed hands.

The paper working surface should lie flat on the trolley top and should never be flattened with the fingers. Forceps are used for removing stitches or for inserting safety pins in drains, otherwise sterile gloved fingers should be used.

Whilst performing an aseptic technique, it is recommended that wherever possible wounds are irrigated using a warm sterile solution, preferably normal saline, and not dried. There is evidence to suggest that cotton wool balls can leave fibres in the wound (Wood, 1976), therefore, if the wound must be cleaned, non-shedding gauze should be used, with each gauze swab used only once and then discarded.

Any sachets containing solutions which are to be used during an aseptic technique should be swabbed at the point of perforation with an alcohol based solution and allowed to air dry prior to use.

Ideally, aseptic procedures should take place in an area where traffic flow is reduced, such as the clinical or treatment room.

4. Procedure for cleaning a trolley for an aseptic technique

Action	Rationale
Ideally, specific trolleys should be kept for use during aseptic procedures only.	This minimises the possibility of contamination of trolleys in the ward area.

Action	Rationale
Trolleys must be prepared and kept in a designated clean area of the ward.	This minimises the possibility of contamination of trolleys in the ward area.
Each day the trolley must be cleaned using detergent and hot water, ensuring the underside of the trolley surfaces are also cleaned, and that no adhesive tape has been left on the trolley legs.	This ensures the trolley is socially clean.
Cleaning must be followed by thorough drying of all surfaces using disposable paper towels.	Drying reduces the risk of micro-organisms multiplying.
Immediately prior to, and following an aseptic procedure, the nurse must ensure that his/her hands are socially clean and the trolley surfaces must be cleaned using an alcohol-based spray or wiped and then dried with paper towels.	This minimises the risk of cross infection by reducing levels of bacteria. It does not make the trolley sterile.
After use the trolley must be cleared of any unused materials and these disposed of in the appropriate way (see Section 5)	

5. Procedure for disposal of equipment

Action	Rationale
After use, clear away trolley and contents, *without* taking trolley into sluice/dirty utility room.	In order to prevent contamination.
Clean the trolley surfaces using an alcohol-based spray or wipe and then dry with paper towels.	To minimise the risk of cross infection.

Used instruments

Instruments supplied by sterile services either accompanying the equipment or supplied separately should be placed in the appropriate bag. This in turn is placed in the ward/department sterile services transportation bag (according to local policy).

Used instruments from a known infected patient are placed in a designated bag appropriately labelled with a biohazard label and transported back to sterile services separately, according to local policy (Department of Health, 1991).

Reuseable equipment

Wherever possible, all disinfection and sterilisation should be carried out by the Central Sterile Supplies Department (CSSD).

Sharps

Refer to local sharps policy for advice on safe disposal of all sharps. The most important points to remember are:

– Disposal of sharps is the responsibility of the user.
– Wherever possible, take the sharps box to the point of use.
– Do not resheath needles by hand.
– If it is necessary to separate the needle from the syringe, use either the sharps box facility or forceps.
– Do not overfill sharps boxes — change when two-thirds full.
– Sharps boxes must be placed in a yellow clinical waste bag prior to transportation.

Intravenous giving sets

Discarded intravenous fluid administration sets are a potential hazard and should be disposed of into a clinical waste bag with the used infusion bag *in situ* to protect the pointed end. If this is impractical, then discarded sets should be placed in the sharps bin for disposal.

N.B. This includes intravenous fluid administration sets used for blood transfusion.

Clinical waste

This category includes soiled surgical dressings, swabs, and other contaminated organic waste, including urinary bags, etc.
All clinical waste *must* be discarded into *yellow* clinical waste bags which must be closed securely. If there is a risk of leakage *two yellow* bags must be used. Heavy gauge bags are provided for theatre use.

6. Sharps policy

Sharps include needles, cannulae, giving sets, scalpels, razor-blades, stitch cutters, broken ampoules and glass. Non-disposable sharps, e.g. specialist needles should be protected before returning to the Central Sterile Supplies Department (CSSD).

Disposal of sharps is the responsibility of the user

40% of needle-stick injuries occur at attempted re-sheathing of needles

Do not re-sheath used needles by hand

Large pieces of broken glass, etc. which are too large to go into a sharps box, should be disposed of separately into a rigid container with other non-combustible material.

Protection measures

Before taking blood, personnel must ensure that their skin is intact. Abrasions and cuts should be covered with waterproof dressings. Gloves are available for added protection.

Sharps in use

To separate a needle from a syringe, use a sharps box facility or forceps whenever possible. The needle must go into the sharps box. The empty syringe can go into the yellow clinical waste bag after routine use. Where blood infection is known or suspected the syringe *must* go into the sharps box.

If it is necessary to re-sheath a needle, on an even surface slide needle into the sheath taking great care. Alternatively, a re-sheathing device can be used to hold a needle sheath.

For blood gas analysis, carefully remove the needle and place blind hub onto syringe for transportation.

Barrels supplied for vacuum blood collection systems are for single use only and must be discarded into a yellow clinical waste bag.

Sharps boxes

Department of Health approved boxes must be provided and used wherever sharps are in use. Wherever possible, take the sharps box to the sharps, *not* the other way round.

Always place the box on an even surface where access is easy and the opening can be seen clearly.

Close the sharps box when it is two thirds full. Do *not* overfill as this could cause damage to users and during transit.

Place no more than two sharps boxes in one yellow clinical waste bag in the designated collection area. If a box is known to contain infected material, a "Danger of Infection" label must be fixed to it.

Accidental injury from sharps

The following are first aid measures which apply to all sharps injuries:

1. Encourage bleeding and flush the injury site under running water. Do *not* suck.
2. Wash the area well with soap and water. Dry and apply waterproof dressing as necessary.

After an injury from a *dirty* sharp, for example contaminated with blood or suspected infected material:

1. Report the injury to the nurse in charge as soon as possible.
2. Contact Occupational Health department as soon as possible for further advice.
3. If a risk of blood-borne infection exists, contact the on-call microbiologist or occupational health personnel via switchboard within 24 hours for advice.
4. Complete an incident form. Include name and identification number of the patient for whom the sharp was used (if known).

References

Bridge W, MacLeod Clark J (1981) Communication in Nursing Care. London: HM & M.

Department of Health (1991) Decontamination of Equipment, Linen or Other Surfaces Contaminated with Hepatitis B and/or Human Immunodeficiency Viruses. London: HMSO.

Finesilver C (1979) Preparation of adult patients for cardiac catheterisation and coronary cineangiography. International Journal of Nursing Studies 15: 211–21.

Lazarus RS, Averill JR (1972) Emotion and Condition in Anxiety: Current Trends in Theory and Research, Vol 1. New York: Academic Press.

Tschudin V (1989) Informed consent. Surgical Nurse 2 (6): 15–17.

United Kingdom Central Council for Nursing, Midwifery and Health Visiting (1992) Code of Professional Conduct. London: UKCC.

Wood RAB (1976) Disintegration of cellulose dressings in open granulating wounds. British Medical Journal 785: 1444–5.

Further Reading

Ayliffe GAJ, Lowbury EJL, Geddes AM, Williams JD (1992) Control of Hospital Infection 3rd edn. London: Chapman and Hall.

Gidley C, (1987) Now wash your hands. Nursing Times 83 (29): 40–2.

Jacobson G et al. (1985) Handwashing: Ring-wearing and number of micro-organisms. Nursing Research 34 (3): 186–8.

Taylor LJ (1978) An evaluation of handwashing techniques. Nursing Times 74 (3): 54–5 and 74 (4): 108–10.

Thomlinson D (1987) "To clean or not to clean?" Nursing Times 35: 71–5

Wilson-Barnett J, Batehup L (1989) Patient Problems: A Research base for Nursing Care. London: Scutari Press.

Chapter 2
First aid treatments following burn injuries

Burns are caused by:

1. Dry heat, e.g. fire or hot objects.
2. Moist heat, e.g. scalds from boiling water or steam.
3. Contact with an electric current or by lightning.
4. Friction, e.g. from a revolving wheel.
5. Strong acids and alkalis, e.g. sulphuric acid or caustic soda.
6. Intense cold, e.g. liquid oxygen, liquid nitrogen or extremely cold metals.
7. Radiation, e.g. exposure to sun or radioactive substances.

Soon after the onset of injury there is an increased risk of infection. Primary shock is not life threatening but in a major burn/scald secondary shock is. The longer a person is in contact with the cause of the injury, the greater that injury will become. For this reason, a first aid procedure is imperative, it can make the difference between a minor, moderate, or major burn, and it can save a life (Kemble and Lamb, 1987).

1. Procedure for the first aid treatment of flame burns

Action	Rationale
If the casualty is inside a building, prevent them from rushing outside.	Movement and/or a breeze from outside will fan the flames and assist with causing more burn trauma to the patient.
Advise the casualty to stop and lay down.	To prevent flames from sweeping upwards (Kemble and Lamb, 1987).
If the room and contents are on fire (or the casualty is in an enclosed space) remove them from the area as quickly as possible whether conscious or not.	Inhalation of toxic or hot gases can be fatal.
Extinguish flames with a coat, curtain, blanket or rug. Hold the blanket in front of yourself for protection and when close enough wrap it tightly around the casualty.	Smothering flames starves them of their oxygen supply and extinguishes them (Marsden, Moffat and Scott, 1992).
Do not use nylon or other flammable material to smother the flames.	This would be like adding fuel to the fire and will cause further burning.

Action	Rationale
Do not roll the casualty along the ground.	This action may cause burning of previously unharmed areas (Marsden, Moffat and Scott, 1992).
Maintain a clear airway.	The individual's ability to breathe clearly throughout should be of major importance.
Cool the burn with water for 10–15 minutes or longer if pain persists and the individual is able to tolerate it.	Water will disperse the heat and minimise the pain and extent of injury to the tissues (Davies 1982; Kinsella and Booth, 1991).
Gently remove rings, watches, belts, shoes, etc., before swelling occurs.	As a result of the burn injury localised swelling will occur. Jewellery may restrict the circulation acting as a tourniquet. Early removal minimises the risk, (Marsden, Moffat and Scott, 1992).
Do not remove adherent burnt clothing.	Clothing will have been rendered sterile by the heat and removal may cause exposure of viable tissue (Marsden, Moffat and Scott, 1992).
Seek medical aid as soon as possible.	To ensure early and appropriate treatment.
Elevate burn injured limbs especially those with circumferential burns.	Minimises swelling of the extremity and constriction of blood vessels which may lead to decreased circulation (Sykes and Bailey, 1975).
Ensure casualty is kept warm with extra clothing or a blanket whilst waiting for medical assistance.	To ease the effect of shock (Kemble and Lamb, 1987).

2 Procedure for the first aid treatment of a scald

Action	Rationale
Remove soaked clothing immediately.	Reduces some of the heat in contact with the skin (Settle, 1986)
Immerse burn-injured area in cold running water for 10–15 minutes, or longer if pain persists and the individual is able to tolerate it.	Minimises pain (Davies, 1982) and reduces tissue damage caused by heat (Lawrence, 1986; Marsden, Moffat and Scott, 1992).
	Prolonged immersion puts the patient at risk of hypothermia (Lawrence, 1987)
If the casualty is a child and will not tolerate having the burn immersed in water, apply non-fluffy, clean material soaked in cool water to the burn-injured area. Talk to the child in a calming manner.	Cool soaks will minimise pain and reduce tissue damage caused by heat (Lawrence, 1986).

Calming the child will help to lessen fear. |

Action	Rationale
Gently remove rings, watches, belts, shoes, etc., before swelling occurs.	As a result of the burn injury, localised swelling will occur. Jewellery may become tight and restrict the circulation acting as a tourniquet. Early removal minimises the risk (Stobert, 1994).
Do not puncture blisters, remove loose skin, etc.	Intact blisters provide a natural protection to damaged tissue. Removal of loose skin can cause pain and contamination of the wound, unless carried out in a suitable environment using an appropriate aseptic technique (Marsden, Moffat and Scott, 1992).
Do not apply lotions, ointments or other agents to the burn injury.	This may cause further pain and damage to burn injured tissue and possible contamination of the wound (Stobert, 1994) and may also impede subsequent examination of the wound (Lawrence, 1987).
Cover the damaged skin with plasticised polyvinylchloride (PVC) — cling film. *Do not* wrap it tightly around the burn injured area.	Cling film acts as a temporary dressing until medical aid is sought. It provides rapid relief from pain (Lendrum and Bowden-Jones, 1976). It is non-adherent and painless on removal (Wilson and French, 1987). However, it can cause constriction to the circulation if wrapped too tightly around a burn injured area. It is readily available in most homes and may be rapidly applied as a first aid measure (Milner, 1988).
If cling film is not available, cover with non-fluffy clean material, such as a linen sheet or pillowcase.	This acts as a temporary cover but may stick to damaged skin and require soaking off on arrival at hospital and may lead to further pain and discomfort for the individual (Marsden, Moffat and Scott, 1992).
Do not use adhesive dressings.	Further pain and damage may be caused to the burn injured area on removal of the dressings.
Do not cover facial burns — leave exposed.	Covering the face may restrict breathing and may cause distress, especially in a child or elderly person.
Seek medical aid as soon as possible.	To ensure early and appropriate treatment.
Elevate all burn injured limbs, especially those with circumferential burns.	Minimises swelling of the extremity and constriction of blood vessels which may lead to decreased circulation (Sykes and Bailey, 1975).
Ensure casualty is kept warm with extra clothing or a blanket whilst waiting for medical assistance.	To ease the effect of shock (Marsden, Moffat and Scott, 1992).

3 Procedure for the first aid treatment of a low voltage electrical burn (domestic supply)

Action	Rationale
Assess the scene and if safe to do so: – Switch off the current – Remove the plug from the electric socket – Wrench the cable free.	To break the circuit between the electrical source and the casualty (Marsden, Moffat and Scott, 1992).
If breaking the contact places you in danger, refrain from doing so. Insulate yourself by standing on a rubber surface, or thick layers of dry cloth, newspapers or a telephone directory.	To protect the first aider from sustaining an electrical injury (Marsden, Moffat and Scott, 1992).
Remove the casualty from the electricity source by pulling away with either a dry rope, wooden stick or by grasping dry clothing.	To move the casualty to a safe area, away from the electrical source (Marsden, Moffat and Scott, 1992).
Do not touch any item which is damp or metallic.	Wet, damp or metallic objects can act as a conductor of electricity. Touching any of these places the first aider in danger (Marsden, Moffat and Scott, 1992).
Assess the casualty for cardiopulmonary arrest, if breathing and/or heartbeat ceases, commence cardiopulmonary resuscitation.	To maintain life support (Marsden, Moffat and Scott, 1992).
Seek medical aid as soon as possible.	To ensure early and appropriate treatment.
Leave all clothing intact but gently remove rings, watches, belts and shoes before swelling occurs.	As a result of the burn injury localised swelling may occur. Jewellery etc., may restrict the circulation acting as a tourniquet. Early removal minimises the risk (Stobert, 1994).
Cover the damaged skin with PVC (cling film).	Cling film acts as a temporary dressing until medical aid is sought. It is non-adherent and painless on removal (Wilson and French, 1987).
If cling film is not available cover with clean non-fluffy material e.g. a linen sheet or pillow-case.	This acts as a temporary dressing but may adhere to damaged skin and cause further pain and discomfort when removed (Marsden, Moffat and Scott, 1992).
Elevate burn-injured limbs (especially those with circumferential burns).	Minimises swelling of the extremity and constriction of blood vessels which may lead to decreased circulation (Sykes and Bailey, 1975).
Ensure casualty is kept warm with extra clothing or a blanket whilst waiting for medical assistance.	To ease the effect of shock, (Marsden, Moffat and Scott, 1992).

4 Procedure for the first aid treatment of a high voltage electrical burn

Action	Rationale
Assess the scene. Initially *Do not* approach closer than 18 metres. Identify whether the casualty has grasped a source of high voltage or not. *Do not* attempt to rescue.	High voltages may jump or arc many metres, physical contact with the electrical source is not necessary to sustain injury (Marsden, Moffat and Scott, 1992).
Switch the electricity supply off, assess the individual for cessation of breathing and heartbeat.	A high voltage electrical shock may cause severe swelling of the airway. Chemical changes may also occur in the nerves, heart and muscles causing the heart to stop (Dimick, 1994).
Commence cardiopulmonary resuscitation (if necessary).	To maintain life support, (Marsden, Moffat and Scott, 1992).
Do not move the individual unless unavoidable.	The individual may have sustained fractured bones and/or dislocation of joints from severe muscle contractions resulting from the burn injury (Dimick, 1994).
Seek medical aid as soon as possible.	To ensure early and appropriate treatment.
Leave all clothing intact but gently remove rings, watches, belts and shoes before swelling occurs.	As a result of the burn injury localised swelling may occur. Jewellery, etc. may restrict the circulation acting as a tourniquet. Early removal minimises the risk (Stobert, 1994).
Cover the damaged skin with PVC (cling film).	Cling film acts as a temporary dressing until medical aid is sought. It is non-adherent and painless on removal, (Wilson and French, 1987).
If cling film is not available cover with clean non-fluffy material, e.g. a linen sheet or pillowcase.	This acts as a temporary dressing but may adhere to damaged skin and cause further pain and discomfort when removed (Marsden, Moffatt and Scott, 1992).
Elevate burn-injured limbs (especially those with circumferential burns).	Minimises swelling of the extremity and constriction of blood vessels which may lead to decreased circulation (Sykes and Bailey, 1975).
Ensure casualty is kept warm with extra clothing or a blanket whilst waiting for medical assistance.	To ease the effect of shock (Marsden, Moffat, and Scott, 1992).

5. Procedure for the first aid treatment of a chemical burn

Action	Rationale
Evaluate the scene. *Do not* give assistance if doing so places you in danger. Seek medical aid immediately.	There may be chemical spillage around or near the casualty and/or toxic fumes may be present (Malem, 1994).
	Trained personnel using the correct equipment can safely apply first aid.
During contact with the casualty, wear rubber or latex gloves (if available).	To protect the first aider from harm (Malem, 1994).
If it is safe to enter the area, dilute the chemical on the skin with gently running water, for at least 20–30 minutes and longer if pain persists. (Irrigation may be required for up to 1 hour in some cases.)	Irrigation with water achieves active dilution and removal of the chemical (Kinsella and Booth, 1991). The active agent will continue to destroy tissue for as long as it remains in contact with the skin, forming a deep ulcer and a progressive lesion (Yano et al., 1993).
	Tissue destruction may occur for up to 72 hours after injury if the chemical is not adequately diluted and removed. Cool water minimises the pain and discomfort for the casualty.
Remove all contaminated clothing and jewellery as irrigation continues.	To reduce the amount of chemical in contact with the skin.
Keep the irrigation procedure under control.	To avoid splashing which may cause further damage.
Avoid powerful shower sprays.	May cause further damage to badly burned tissue and result in additional pain and discomfort for the casualty.
Ensure the water drains away freely and safely.	The water will be contaminated by the chemical and may cause further damage if collecting in a pool.
N.B. Exceptions — If the chemical is dry such as lime:	Mixing dry lime and water creates a corrosive liquid which may cause further tissue damage (Wilson and Davidson, 1985).
– Brush any dry chemical from the casualty's skin, hair and clothing.	To facilitate removal of the chemical.
– Remove any contaminated clothing as soon as possible.	
– Avoid contaminating the eyes and the airway.	To minimise damage to the eyesight and minimise risk of respiratory distress.

Action	Rationale
– Irrigate the skin as above.	To facilitate removal of the chemical.
Seek medical aid as soon as possible.	To ensure early and appropriate treatment.
Cover the injured part with non-fluffy clean material, e.g. a linen sheet or pillowcase, or PVC (cling film).	Cling film acts as a temporary dressing until medical aid is sought. It is non-adherent and painless on removal (Wilson and French, 1987).
The appropriate neutralising agent may be sought only after initial, immediate, water irrigation and medical aid has been called for.	A neutralising agent used at an early stage can produce heat by interacting with the chemical and may cause further tissue damage.
	Time is wasted identifying the chemical and neutralising agent. Water irrigation can be carried out immediately, thus decreasing the rate of reaction between the tissue and the active agent (Marsden, Moffat and Scott, 1992).

To obtain further information on antidotes contact:

1. Queens Medical Centre, A & E Department.   0115 9249924
Reception, Ext 43671
or 43675

2. National Chemical Emergency Centre, Oxfordshire.   01235 24141
Ext 2121

3. Guy's Hospital Poison Centre, London.   0171 635 9191
or 0171 407 7600

6. Procedure for the first aid treatment of a tar burn (e.g. bitumen)

Action	Rationale
Ensure airways are clear.	If tar has spilled over the head and face the casualty may not be able to breathe normally.
Cool the injured part with cold running water for 10–30 minutes.	As long as the tar is hot, tissue destruction continues. Cooling will minimise pain and discomfort (Marsden, Moffat and Scott, 1992).
Leave bitumen adherent to the skin and cover with PVC (cling film).	Bitumen itself will act as a temporary dressing until removed. Cling film minimises spread of tar onto clothes, etc. and acts as a non-stick temporary dressing (Wilson and French, 1985).
Seek medical aid as soon as possible.	To ensure immediate and appropriate treatment.

Action	Rationale
Apply baby oil, mineral oil, butter or petroleum jelly to the affected area.	Baby oil (Juma, 1994), mineral oil, such as eucalyptus oil, butter (Tiernan and Harris, 1993) or petroleum jelly will aid removal of tar. However, the removal will need to be carried out within a suitable environment and by qualified personnel.

References

Davies JWL (1982) Prompt cooling of burned areas — A review of the benefits and the effector mechanisms, Burns Journal 9: 1–6.

Dimick R (1994) Electrical injuries. In: Harrison TR, (Ed) Principles of International Medicine. 13th ed New York: McGraw-Hill. pp 2480–2.

Juma A (1994) Bitumen burns and the use of baby oil. Journal of the International Society for Burn Injuries 20 (4): 363–5.

Kemble JVH, Lamb B (1987) Practical Burns Management. London: Hodder and Stoughton. pp 18–22.

Kinsella J, Booth MG (1991) Pain-relief in burns. James Laing Memorial Essay 1990. Burns Journal 17 (5): 391–5.

Lawrence JC, Wilkins MD (1986) The epidemiology of burns. In (Ed) Burn Care — A Teaching Symposium. Hull: Smith and Nephew.

Lawrence JC (1987) British Burn Association. Recommended first aid for burns and scalds. Burns Journal 13 (2): 153.

Lendrum J, Bowden-Jones E, (1976) A new dressing for burns. Enclosure in a plasticised polyvinyl sheet. Burns Journal 2: 86.

Malem F (1994) Nurse-aid management of casualties of hazardous substances. British Journal of Nursing 3 (8): 425–8.

Marsden AK, Moffat C, Scott R (1992) First Aid Manual. London: Dorling Kindersley.

Milner RH (1988) Plasticised polyvinyl-chloride film as temporary burns dressing — A Microbiological Study. Burns Journal 14 (1): 62–5.

Settle JAD (1986) Burns the First Five Days. Essex: Smith and Nephew

Stobert L (1994) Nurse-aid management of burns. British Journal of Nursing 3 (9): 469–72.

Sykes PJ, Bailey BN (1975) Treatment of hand burns with occlusive bags. A comparison of three methods. Burns Journal 2: 163.

Tiernan E, Harris A (1993) Butter in the initial treatment of hot tar burns. Journal of the International Society for Burn Injuries. 19 (5): 437–8.

Wilson GR, Davidson PM (1985) Full thickness burns from ready mixed cement. Journal of the International Society for Burn Injuries. 19 (5): 437–8.

Wilson G, French G (1987) Plasticised polyvinyl-chloride as a temporary dressing for burns. British Medical Journal 294: 556–7.

Yano K, Hata Y, Matsuka K, Ito O, Matsuda H (1993) Experimental study on alkaline skin injuries — Periodic changes in subcutaneous tissue pH and the effects exerted by washing. Journal of the International Society for Burn Injuries 19 (4): 320–3.

Further Reading

Lawrence C, (1989) Treating minor burns. Nursing Times 85: 69–73.

Muir IFK, Barclay TL, Settle JAD (1987) Burns and their Treatment London: Butterworth. pp 142–5.

Chapter 3
Wound care following burn trauma

A burn can be caused by scalds, flames, chemicals, electricity, or radiation. Prompt and appropriate first aid treatment at the moment of burning and in the ensuing few minutes after injury may make the difference between a major, moderate or minor burn injury (Kemble and Lamb, 1987).

The ability of the skin to repair itself is dependent on the depth of skin damage which is an important factor in deciding the outcome of a burn and how it is managed (see Figure 3.1).

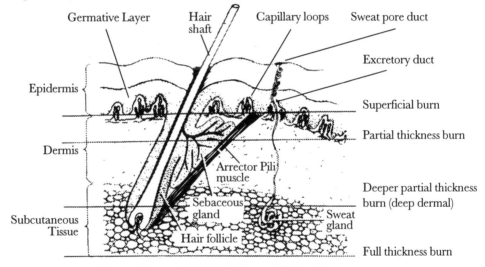

Figure 3.1 *The structure of the skin showing the depth of skin damage following burn trauma.*

Superficial burns involve loss of the epidermis only. The epithelium repairs itself very efficiently by mitosis and cell migration and usually heals in 7–10 days (Muddiman, 1989).

Partial thickness burns involve loss of the epidermis and the superficial layers of the dermis. Providing some dermal cells remain they will regenerate and extend out over the wound to provide complete skin cover. Such wounds should heal uneventfully within 14–21 days by the growth of epithelium from surviving foci provided by the undamaged shafts of hair follicles and sweat ducts deep in the dermis of the burn (Lawrence, 1989).

Deeper partial thickness (deep dermal) burns involve total loss of the epidermis and a significant amount of the dermis. Healing is prolonged with poor skin quality. Better results can be obtained with skin grafting.

Full thickness burns involve total loss of the whole thickness of the dermis. These wounds heal only by regeneration of the dermal cells around the edges of the burn and may take months to heal, leaving a fragile scar. The recommended treatment is therefore closure of the wounds with skin grafts (Lawrence, 1989).

Since infection of the burn wound and its sequelae are responsible for the majority of fatalities following burn trauma, treatment of the wound is directed towards minimising the colonisation of the wound with organisms. Any dead tissue provides an excellent medium for bacteria to multiply, therefore frequent wound debridement using strict aseptic techniques until all necrotic tissue has been removed is an important aspect of wound care and frequent monitoring of the wound surface by bacteriological swabbing is essential.

Treatment

In superficial or partial thickness burns, irrigate the area with water or saline. If blisters are present puncture and expel the fluid then gently remove any loose or dead epithelium with metal forceps and sterile scissors (Rockwell and Ehrlich, 1990). Clip any hair in the surrounding area to minimise the risk of infection. For small areas apply a hydrocolloid dressing, for larger areas apply two or more layers of paraffin gauze and cover with cotton gauze, Gamgee and bandage. Reassess the wound every 2–3 days. (Burns to the face can be left exposed providing the atmosphere is clean, warm and dry. Exudate is removed frequently using water or saline). The aim of the treatment is to provide a moist environment to promote migration of epithelium, to protect the burn wound surface from infection or injury, and to absorb excess exudate.

In deep dermal or full thickness burns the wounds are best skin grafted early before the loose or dead epithelium can become colonised by bacteria. When the patient's condition is stable and the burn wound is relatively free from pathogenic bacteria, the eschar is surgically excised down to healthy tissue and covered with a skin graft (Konop, 1991).

If early excision is not possible the burn wound is irrigated with water, saline or povidone iodine, and frequent wound debridement should be carried out. The burns are treated using either an enzymatic treatment to assist with debridement, e.g. Varidase, or a hydrogel product, e.g. Intrasite, or an antibacterial agent, e.g. Silver sulphadiazine cream and covered with secondary dressings, e.g. layers of cotton gauze, Gamgee and bandage. (It is important that dressings are thick enough to exclude ingress of organisms from the environment and allow for absorption of excess exudate). Reassess the wound every 2–3 days. The aim of the treatment is to control the proliferation of bacteria on the burn wound surface, to provide a moist environment, to encourage the separation of burn eschar, and to debride the area to achieve a clean vascularised wound which will accept a skin graft.

Management of burn wounds

The management of burn wounds continues to be an area of extensive debate and research (Queen et al., 1987; Monafo and Freedman, 1987; Lloyd and Mickel, 1989; Dziewulski, 1992; Wright, MacKechnie and Paskins, 1993; Gower and Lawrence, 1995). Burn wounds require a thorough and accurate assessment to determine depth, percentage body surface area involved, progression or regression in wound healing, evidence of clinical infection, and the most appropriate choice of wound care product.

Whether using an aseptic or socially clean technique for wound care the nurse should have a good working knowledge of the principles of infection control. Aseptic technique involves using sterile objects and fluids whilst minimising the risk of airborne contamination (Aycliffe et al.,1992). A non-touch technique requires the use of sterile gloves or forceps within a sterile field. Using the correct technique can contribute to the healing process (Lascelles, 1982). Using gloves for wound care is recommended rather than forceps since the latter may impair manual dexterity and cause tissue damage and pain (Glide, 1992).

Using cotton wool for cleaning enhances the risk of the material shedding fibres into a wound and disrupts the healing process (Wood, 1976). The fibres may also act as a foreign body and provide a focus for infection (Thomas, 1990). Foam, sponges or non-woven gauze are recommended alternatives.

Solutions used for wound irrigation or cleansing should be warmed to body temperature prior to use, to minimise any delays in wound healing caused by a drop in wound surface temperature (Turner, 1985; Lock, 1980). Saline is the most desirable solution as it is non-toxic, has no side-effects, and is cheap and cost effective. Irrigation is preferable to cleaning a wound as cleaning may damage new epithelium and is painful for the patient (Glide, 1992). Irrigation is more effective and less harmful in the long term (Thomas, 1990).

The ideal burn wound dressing must protect the wound from physical damage and micro-organisms, be comfortable, compliant, durable, non-toxic, non-adherent, non-irritant, compatible with toxic therapeutic agents, and be able to produce a wound environment that permits healing to occur as rapidly as possible (Lawrence, 1983).

Burn wound dressings

It is widely accepted that burns require dressings. In the UK the use of dressing products combined with topical antibacterial agents is one of the desired methods of treatment (Lawrence, 1989).

All burns contain dead tissue which forms an excellent bacterial culture medium and puts the patient at risk from infection. Therefore, isolating the wound from the environment and using topical antibacterial therapy is frequently practised. Antibacterial agents suitable for use in burn wound management are limited, with Silver Sulphadiazine being one of the most widely used (Hamilton-Miller, Shah and Smith, 1993).

Absorbent wool dressings may be used. However, they lose their bacterial barrier properties in the presence of moisture. Leakage from the wound, slippage and pain merit prompt dressing removal and wound inspection (Lawrence, 1989).

Paraffin gauze is widely used as a primary wound contact layer together with absorbent gauze, secured by crepe bandage. It is unwise to use tulles containing antibiotics because of the risk of the emergence of resistant bacterial strains.

Various creams can also be used to treat burns in combination with traditional dressings but these may be expensive.

Several of the more modern dressing materials can be used as alternatives to conventional products. Semi-permeable adhesive films and hydrocolloid dressings may enhance the healing time of burns and have the advantage of being waterproof and less bulky.

Each patient should be assessed on an individual basis and the nurse should demonstrate an extensive knowledge of wound care products in order choose the most appropriate treatment.

1. Procedure for the isolation of patients on the Burns Unit

There are two types of isolation on the Burns Unit: protective and source.
Protective isolation is indicated for:

1. Patients following major burn trauma from admission to skin cover.
2. Patients with facial burns.
3. Patients with perineal burns which are exposed.
4. Patients more at risk of infection as a result of drug therapy, age or poor general physical condition.

Source isolation is indicated to:

1. Minimise the spread of infection to other patients and staff.
2. Isolate specific types of infections, e.g. Beta Haemolytic Streptococcus groups A, B, C, G, and Methicillin Resistant *Staphylococcus Aureus* (MRSA).

See sections 1 and 2 in Chapter 1 for advice on procedures.

Equipment

Unsterile gloves
Plastic aprons
Antiseptic soap (4% chlorhexidine glyconate)
Alcohol hand-rub solution
Sharps box
Advice sheet
Mop and bucket

Action	Rationale
Inform senior nurse in infection control either via telephone, or Burns Unit link nurse if the patient requires source isolation.	To seek suitable advice and to maintain statistical information records.
Prepare the designated room as soon as possible. – Switch the heating up (if cool). – Remove any equipment not required. – Stock up with adequate supplies of gloves, aprons, antiseptic soap and/or alcohol hand-rub solution and a sharps box.	To ensure the wearing of necessary protective clothing, and effective handwashing for all necessary procedures (Wilson, 1992).
N.B. Utilise specific single rooms on the unit if source isolation is required, keeping isolation period to a minimum.	Specific rooms are designated as source isolation rooms with double doors and toilet facilities en-suite. Sensory input associated with isolation can have serious psychological effects on the patient (Denton, 1986).
If source isolation is required, promptly inform relevant staff on the unit including domestic staff. Request mop and bucket for individual use in the single room.	To maintain awareness of the situation with domestic staff and to allow provision of mop and bucket for individual use in the single room.
Isolate the patient in the designated single room.	Provision of single room facilities allows isolation of the source of the infection, allows dressing changes to be performed in a closed environment minimising the spread of infection through dust and/or skin particles and reduces the amount of unnecessary visits to the patient. It can also be used for the protection of the patient (Wilson, 1992).
Ask the infection control nurse to complete an advice sheet for the patient if source isolation is required.	For clear instructions and guidance on disposal of linen, rubbish, crockery, sharps, CSSD and care of toilet facilities.

Action	Rationale
Inform the medical staff if isolating a patient with a specific type of infection.	With some types of infection the patient may require antibiotic therapy to be prescribed.
Educate staff and the patient's visitors on the strict use of wearing aprons and gloves when in contact with the patient and strict handwashing in between.	Most bacterial contamination is at the front of uniforms (Babb et al., 1983). Using plastic aprons when in contact with the patient minimises the risk of cross infection (Hambreus, 1973).
Damp dust all surfaces in the room daily using detergent and hot water and dry thoroughly (Keep equipment to a minimum.)	To prevent an accumulation of dust which may harbour micro-organisms. Damp dusting assists in maintaining low levels of cross infection (Caddow, 1989). Damp dusting is pointless if thorough drying is not performed, as airborne bacteria colonise on wet surfaces (Caddow, 1989). The recommended cleaning agent for damp dusting is ordinary household detergent (Hills, 1982).
	To maximise use of equipment for all patients on the unit.
Take bacteriological wound swabs for culture and sensitivity at each dressing change, label and send to microbiology.	To detect early signs of infection or to monitor when the patient is clear from infection.
Record in the appropriate documentation.	To maintain an accurate record.
N.B. For advice on cleaning the room and equipment after discharge, refer to local infection control guidelines.	For clear instructions and guidance.

References

Aycliffe GAJ, Lowbury EJL, Geddes AM, Williams JD (1992) Control of Hospital Infection 3rd Ed. London: Chapman and Hall.

Babb JR, et al. (1983) Contamination protective clothing and nurses uniforms in an isolation ward. Journal of Hospital Infection 4: 149–57.

Caddow P (1989) Applied Microbiology Middlesex: Scutari Press. p 87.

Denton PF (1986) Psychological and physiological effects of isolation. Nursing 3 (4): 88–91.

Dziewulski P (1992) Burn wound healing — James Ellsworth Laing Memorial Essay for 1991. Journal of the International Society for Burn Injuries 18 (6): 466–78.

Glide S (1992) Cleaning choices. Nursing Times 88 (19): 74–8.

Gower JP, Lawrence JC (1995) The incidence, cause and treatment of minor burns. Journal of Wound Care 4 (2): 71–4.

Hambreus A (1973) Transfer of *Staphylococcus Aureus* via nurses uniforms. Journal of Hygiene 71: 799–814.

Hamilton-Miller JMT, Shah S, Smith C (1993) Silver sulphadiazine — A comprehensive *in vitro* reassessment. Chemotherapy 39: 405–9.

Hills S (1982) Which disinfectants do nurses use? Nursing Times 80 (7): 60–1.

Kemble HJV, Lamb B (1987) Practical Burns Management. London: Hodder and Stoughton.

Konop DJ (1991) General local treatment. In: Trofino RB (Ed.) Nursing Care of the Burn Injured Patient. Philadelphia: FA Davis Company. pp 42–67.

Lascelles I (1982) Wound dressing techniques. Nursing 2nd Series 2 (8): 217–19.

Lawrence JC (1983) Laboratory studies of dressings. Cited in Wound Healing Turner TD, (1985) Which Dressing and Why. In: Westaby S (Ed) Wound Care. London: Heinemann.

Lawrence JC (1989) Management of Burns. The Dressing Times 2 (3): 1–4.

Lloyd DA, Mickel RE (1989) Tropical treatment of burns using aserbine. Burns Journal 15 (2): 125–8.

Lock P (1980) Proceedings of the Symposium of Wound Healing. Gothenburg: Linden and Somer.

Monafo WW, Freedman B, (1987) Topical therapy for burns. Surgical Clinics of North America. 67: 133

Muddiman R (1989) A new concept in hand burn dressings. Nursing Standard Special Supplement: pp 1–30.

Queen D, Evans JH, Gaylor JDS, Courtney JM, Reid WH (1987) Burn wound dressings. A review. Burns Journal 13 (3): 218–28.

Rockwell WB, Ehrlich HP (1990) Should burn blisters be burst? Journal of Burn Care and Rehabilitation 11: 93.

Thomas S (1990) Wound Management and Dressings. London: Pharmaceutical Press.

Turner TD (1985) 1 Which Dressing and Why. In: Westby S, (Ed) Wound Care. London: Heinemann.

Wilson J (1992) Theory and practice of isolation. Nursing Standard 6 (17): 30–1.

Wood RAB (1976) Disintegration of cellulose dressings in open granulating wounds. British Medical Journal. 12 June: 1444–5.

Wright A, MacKechnie DWM, Paskins JR (1993) Management of partial thickness burns with Granuflex E dressings. Journal of the International Society for Burn Injuries 19 (2): 128–130.

Further Reading

Gould D, Chamberlain A (1994) Gram negative bacteria. The challenge of preventing cross infection in hospital wards. A review of the literature. Journal of Clinical Nursing 3: 339–45.

Porter M (1992) Making sense of dressings. Journal of Wound Management 2 (2): 10–12.

Chapter 4
Care of a patient with burns to the eye

A burn injury to the eye can occur as a result of intense heat, chemicals, contact, electrical/laser equipment, or X-rays. The resulting damage can affect the eyelid, conjunctiva, cornea and/or the deeper, surrounding tissues. In some cases the injury may be severe enough to cause infections, contractures of the eyelid, corneal ulceration and even loss of vision (Sadowski, 1991). See Figure 4.1 for the anatomy of the eye.

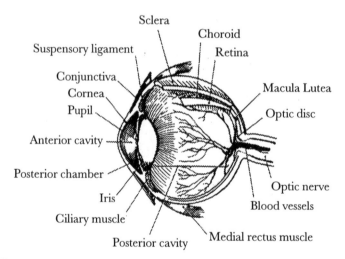

Figure 4.1 *The anatomy of the eye. (From Watson's Medical-Surgical Nursing and Related Physiology 4th Ed (1992) (Eds) Royal JA, Walsh M reproduced with permission from Baillière Tindall).*

The extent of injury to the eyelid can be minor, moderate or major.

1. Minor: A superficial or partial thickness burn may be wet, sensitive to touch and with blister formation in some cases. Usually heals in 5–7 days.
2. Moderate: A deeper partial thickness burn which is painful and results in oedema formation shortly after the burn injury. (The formation of oedema is an advantage to the patient as it keeps the eye moist and prevents further damage.) Usually heals without surgical intervention.
3. Major: A deep partial thickness or full thickness burn is usually associated with contracture and ectropion of the eyelid. As the lid is unable to close the cornea dries and becomes ulcerated.

Chemical

Chemical burns may be classified as toxic, acid or alkaline (Rozenbaum, Baruchin and Dafna, 1991). Acid burns are usually self-contained; however, alkaline burns cause more extensive damage and ocular impairment. The damage may include opacity or ulceration of the cornea, keratinisation of the conjunctiva with glaucoma and cataracts developing at a later stage. The severity of the injury depends on the concentration of the chemical, the toxity and the duration of contact (Hughes, 1946; Grant, 1974).

Substances such as lime (CaO) cause more damage than acids (Pavan-Langston, 1985) because of their rapid penetration through the cornea and the anterior chamber. Damage is related to the pH, the higher the pH the more significant the damage to the eye especially around pH 11 (Grant, 1974).

The immediate care is to irrigate the eye with copious amounts of water or saline to dilute the chemical. Eversion of the upper eyelid may need to be performed to ensure all surfaces have been adequately irrigated. Analgesia may be added to relieve pain and the patient should be referred to an ophthalmologist promptly (Rozenbaum, Baruchin and Dafna, 1991).

Contact

Contact burns may result from hot flying objects, e.g. molten metal, or from direct contact, e.g. the lighted tip of a cigarette or cigar. The severity will depend on the duration of contact, the heat intensity and the area of contact (Sadowski, 1991).

The patient will immediately complain of pain, blurred vision, continuous watering of the eyes and photophobia. The eye should be irrigated with water or saline to decrease the heat and examined to detect any foreign bodies which will need to be removed.

Electrical

Damage may not be revealed for several months after the initial injury (Sadowski, 1991). The incidence is higher in patients who have sustained electrical burns to the head and/or neck.

Flash

In a flash injury the eyes are protected by the blink reflex and the cornea is rarely involved. It is essential to examine the eyes, especially if there is a history of being injured in an enclosed space. If there are any signs of corneal injury then the assistance of an ophthalmologist should be sought (Guy et al., 1994).

Where there is no evidence of burn trauma to the eyelids, this may imply that the eyes were open at the time of exposure to the thermal energy and corneal burns may be present.

Assessment of ocular burns requires inspection of the lid, both fornices, and the globe, and testing of the level of visual acuity. The cornea should be examined for oedema, the iris for opacity due to protein coagulation, and the conjunctiva for hyperaemia and epithelial loss. In severe injuries there may be ischaemia of the sclera and loss of vascularity. Examination of the eye should also include observing for globe penetration and evidence of foreign bodies.

Corneal burns have been classified into four grades by Ealing and Roper-Hall (1986). Treatment following initial irrigation of the globe is directed towards minimising infection and promoting healing with minimal scarring.

1. Procedure for the care of a patient with burns to the eye on admission to the Burns Unit

See sections 1 and 2 in Chapter 1 for advice on procedures.

Equipment

Clean tray
Fluorescein eye drops
Ophthalmoscope or ultraviolet lamp
500ml bag of 0.9% saline and intravenous administration set (optional)
Water-repellent sheet
Disposable gloves
Clean bowl or jug
Patient's prescription chart
Nursing documentation charts

Action	Rationale
On admission of the patient to the Burns Unit, obtain a detailed history of the injury, e.g. cause and duration of contact.	To assist in ascertaining the severity of the injury. History allows for appropriate interventions to be performed.
Ask the patient if contact lenses are worn.	To determine whether these will need to be removed.
Ask the patient if they have any pain, noting quality and intensity. Administer analgesia as prescribed by the medical staff.	To minimise pain and discomfort for the patient. Eye burns are generally painful (Frank, Wachtel and Frank, 1983) and adequate analgesia is required to minimise pain and discomfort for the patient.
Observe the patient for signs of visual disturbances, itchiness around the eyes and/or photophobia.	To detect early signs of complications.

Action	**Rationale**
Perform a physical inspection of the eyes:	To assist with assessing and evaluating any damage to the eyes and in determining any appropriate action. Also indicates evidence of ocular damage (Sadowski, 1991).
– Observe for singed eyelashes and eyebrows. – Observe the eyelids for abrasions, lacerations, bleeding, oedema and ability to close. – Observe conjunctiva for lacerations, abrasions, colour and foreign bodies. – Observe the cornea for opacity. – Observe the pupils for size, shape, equality and reaction to light.	Opacity may affect vision Semidilated and/or fixed pupils may signify a chemical injury (Saini and Sharma, 1993).
If a chemical injury is suspected and first aid treatment has been limited:	
– Drape the water-repellent sheet around the patient's shoulders. – Irrigate the eye by attaching an intravenous administration set to a 500 ml bag of 0.9% saline for 20–30 minutes.	Irrigation for 20–30 minutes will dilute and flush out the chemical from the eye (Sadowski, 1991; Rozenbaum, Baruchin and Dafna, 1991) limiting severity of the injury and reducing ocular morbidity (Saini and Sharma, 1993).
– Place the end of the tubing across the bridge of the nose pointed towards the inner canthus of the eye and allow the fluid to run across the eye diluting and flushing out any chemical deposits that may be remaining into a bowl or jug.	Directing the fluid towards the outer canthus may cause the chemical to penetrate deeper into the eye rather than flushing it out and may also splash onto the other eye.
Prior to examination of the eye by the medical staff instil 1–2 drops of fluorescein into the eye. Wait a few seconds then examine the eye using an ophthalmoscope or ultraviolet lamp.	Fluorescein temporarily stains the eye. When examined through the ophthalmoscope or using an ultraviolet lamp any damage to the cornea and/or conjunctiva will be evident (Sadowski, 1991).
For extensive injuries refer the patient to an opthalmologist.	For a more detailed assessment and advice on treatment.

2. Procedure for eye care

Eyes are initially examined by both medical and nursing staff as part of the admission procedure before oedema of the eyelids occurs. Burns patients require regular effective eye care because:

1. Damage to the eyelids may prevent closure of the eyes, e.g. as a result of deeper or full thickness burns.

2. Corneal abrasions may occur as a result of debris in the eye or drying of the cornea if the eyelids are unable to close.
3. Crusting occurs when the eyelids do not move normally.
4. Patients may be unable to care for their own eyes.
5. Slough or eschar on the eyelids may cause infection.

See sections 1 and 2 in Chapter 1 for advice on procedures.

Equipment

Trolley or tray
Sterile eye dressing pack
Sachet of normal saline and alcohol swab
Disposable gloves
Small sterile gauze swabs
Hypromellose eye drops and/or prescribed eye drops/ointment
Patient's prescription chart

Action	Rationale
Help the patient into a comfortable position.	To maintain the comfort of the patient.
Assess the condition of the patient's eyes	To determine the appropriate treatment required.
Prepare the eye pack and apply gloves.	To minimise the risk of cross infection.
Identify one hand per eye or treat one eye completely then change gloves and repeat the procedure for the other eye.	To minimise the risk of cross infection.
Request or help the patient to close the eyes.	To minimise the risk of corneal damage during the procedure.
Moisten the sterile gauze swabs with saline.	Moistened gauze will facilitate easier removal of discharge or crusts from around the eye (Sadowski, 1991). Cotton wool should be avoided as any threads left *in situ* may provide a medium for the growth of organisms (Wood, 1976).
Wipe the eyelids gently from the nose outwards using each gauze swab once only.	To clean the eyelid and minimise the risk of cross infection.
If both lids are damaged, wipe each separately asking the patient to look upwards or downwards accordingly.	Assists with more thorough cleansing and minimises the risk of cross infection.

Action	Rationale
Dry the eyes gently using the gauze swabs. Care must be taken not to wipe across the cornea.	To minimise the risk of corneal damage during the procedure.
Instil one hypromellose drop into each eye.	To hydrate the eye and reduce the risk of keratitis (Muir, Barclay and Settle, 1987).
– With one finger retract the lower lid (hold the dropper in the other hand). – Ask the patient to look upwards. – Allow one drop to fall onto the centre of the lining of the lower lid from about 2 cm above the eye.	To facilitate efficient application of the eye drops.
– If possible ask the patient to close the eyelids for 30 seconds and then blink several times.	To encourage dispersion of the drop allowing the solution to pass over the whole of the eye.
Instil prescribed ophthalmic antibiotic drops as above or apply prescribed ophthalmic antibiotic ointment.	Decreases the risk of tissue irritation and infection (Sadowski, 1991).
– With one finger retract the lower lid (hold the tube in other hand). – Ask the patient to look upwards. – Squeeze approximately 1 cm of ointment into the centre of the lining of the lower lid. **N.B. In patients with severe oedema to the eyelids and who may be unable to open the eyes *DO NOT* retract the lower lid but squeeze the ointment as close as possible along the line of the eyelashes.**	To facilitate efficient application of the eye ointment.
Request or help the patient to close the eyes and using the gauze swabs, gently wipe away any excess fluid or ointment.	To protect the cornea, whilst wiping away excess medication and for the comfort of the patient.
N.B. Do not cover the eyes. Remove gloves and wash hands.	The eyes should not be covered as corneal abrasions can occur (Sadowski, 1991).
Repeat the procedure 2–4 hourly or more frequently as required.	To maintain effective removal of discharge or crusts (Sadowski, 1991).
Record administration of drops or ointment on the prescription chart and record procedure in the appropriate documentation.	To maintain an accurate record.

Action	Rationale
Assess the involved eye every 2 hours for blurriness, pain, conjunctivitis and/or corneal drying, tearing, drainage, oedema, tenderness, redness and reaction to light.	Determines changes as they are occurring allowing for appropriate therapeutic interventions to be performed (Sadowski, 1991).
Record in the appropriate documentation.	To maintain an accurate record.

References

Ealing EM, Roper-Hall KJ (1986) Eye Injuries: An Illustrated Guide. London: Butterworths.

Frank DH, Wachtel T, Frank HA (1983) The early treatment and reconstruction of eyelid burns. Journal of Trauma 23 (10): 874.

Grant WM (1974) Toxicology of the Eye. 2nd Ed Springfield Illanois: Thomas. pp 8–101.

Guy PR, Taggart I, Adeniran A, Burd DA (1994) Corneal burns with eyelid sparing and their treatment. Journal of the International Society for Burn Injuries 20 (6): 561–3.

Hughes EF (1946) Alkali burns of the eye. Review of the literature and summary of present knowledge. Archives of Opthalmology 36: 189.

Muir IFK, Barclay TL, Settle JAD (1987) Burns and Their Treatment 3rd Ed. London: Butterworths.

Pavan-Langston D (Ed) (1985) Burns and trauma. Cited in Manual of Ocular Diseases and Therapy. Boston: Little Brown.

Rozenbaum D, Baruchin AM, Dafna Z (1991) Chemical burns of the eye with special reference to alkali burns. Journal of the International Society for Burn Injuries 17 (2): 136–9.

Sadowski DA (1991) Burns of the eyes and ears. In Trofino RB, (Ed) Nursing Care of the Burn Injured Patient. Philadelphia: FA Davis. pp 184–201.

Saini JS, Sharma A (1993) Ocular chemical burns clinical and demographic profile. Journal of the International Society for Burn Injuries 19 (1): 67–9.

Wood RAB (1976) Disintegrating of cellulose dressings in open granulating wounds. British Medical Journal 785: 1444 -5.

Chapter 5
Care of a patient with burns to the ear

A burn injury to the ears can occur as a result of direct thermal injury. The resulting damage may occur as a deep partial thickness (deep dermal) or full thickness burn (Sadowski, 1991). In the event of a deep partial thickness burn cartilage may not be directly exposed but because of oedema formation and the contracture caused by the overlying eschar there may be a decrease in vascularity resulting in necrosis of the underlying cartilage (Dowling, Foley and Moncrief, 1968; Goel, Law and MacMillan, 1983). With a full thickness burn there is an immediate lack of blood supply to the cartilage leading to necrosis of the tissue (Sadowski, 1991). Treatment is aimed at maintaining a moist environment to promote wound healing, applying topical antibacterial agents or desloughing agents and allowing the eschar to separate spontaneously rather than initiating prompt surgical intervention.

Burns to the ears can result in an infection known as chondritis which manifests itself 2–6 weeks post burn injury. The patient will complain of pain and tenderness in the affected ear and it gradually becomes red, warm to touch and oedematous. Inflammation may occur over the whole of the ear and purulent drainage may also be observed (Sadowski, 1991). Treatment is to commence antibiotic therapy, incise and drain any abscess formation, remove dead cartilage and avoid external pressure on the ears by dressings or pillows to minimise pain. Despite prompt action severe ear deformity or loss of the ear may occur (Engrau, 1987).

Because of the oedema formation that can occur with burns to the ears the patient may experience some hearing deficit. It is important to coordinate with the patient a communication system to minimise fear and anxiety and to assist with orientation to the environment if hearing loss occurs.

Ear burns can cause severe pain. Analgesia should be prescribed by the medical staff and administered regularly and the effectiveness continually monitored to minimise the pain and discomfort experienced by the patient.

1. Procedure for the care of a patient with burns to the ears on admission to the Burns Unit

See sections 1 and 2 in Chapter 1 for advice on procedures.

Equipment

Clean tray
Auriscope
Disposable gloves
PVC (cling film)
Patient's prescription chart
Nursing documentation charts

Action	Rationale
On admission of the patient obtain a detailed history of the injury, e.g. cause and duration of contact with the source.	To assist in ascertaining the severity of the injury. History allows for appropriate interventions to be performed (Sadowski, 1991).
Determine if any first aid treatment was undertaken and which type of ointments and/or temporary dressings were applied.	To assess whether appropriate interventions have been performed.
Check if the patient wears any hearing aids and if so, who has possession of them.	To determine whether the patient has a previous hearing impairment (Sadowski, 1991).
Ask the patient if they have any pain, its quality and intensity. Administer analgesia as prescribed by the medical staff.	Ear burns can cause severe pain, analgesia will minimise pain and discomfort for the patient (Sadowski, 1991).
Frequently ask the patient if any difficulty in hearing or any ringing/buzzing in the ears is being experienced.	Hearing may be distorted, partially or totally, by the injury. Ongoing assessments determine if any abnormalities are improving, stabilising or progressing (Sadowski, 1991).
Perform a physical inspection of the ears:	To assist with determining and evaluating the severity of burns to the ears and in determining any appropriate action to be taken.
– Examine the auricles for any deformities, lesions, pain or drainage.	
– Assess any drainage for type, amount, and colour.	If the drainage is bright red, internal bleeding may be suspected (Sadowski, 1991).
– Observe for any signs of tenderness, redness or inflammation.	To detect for early signs of infection (Sadowski, 1991).
– Inspect the ear canal for any discharge, oedema, foreign bodies, redness or abrasions.	Bleeding may signify serious damage and should be dealt with promptly (Sadowski, 1991).

Action	Rationale
Cover the ear with PVC (cling film).	To act as a temporary dressing until the medical staff can assess the ear (Wilson and French, 1985).
For extensive injuries, refer the patient to the ENT department.	For a more detailed assessment and advice on treatment.
Record history and physical examination in the appropriate documentation.	To maintain an accurate record.

2. Procedure for the care of burns to the ears

A burn injury to the pinna of the ear is not an uncommon occurrence with burns to the face and neck. Because of the anatomical position, poor vascularity, the obvious lack of subcutaneous tissue and the superficial location of the cartilage, burns to the ear may result in deeper partial thickness (deep dermal) or full thickness burns. As a result, burns of the ear require prompt attention and treatment. Dressings are aimed at patient comfort, maintaining a moist environment to assist with the promotion of healing, and to minimise the risk of infection.

See sections 1–5 in Chapter 1 for advice on procedures.

Equipment

Trolley
Sterile dressing pack
Sachet of normal saline and alcohol swab
1 pair of unsterile gloves
1 pair of sterile gloves
Sterile gauze swabs
Topical antibacterial cream
Paraffin gauze
Sterile towel
Bacteriological wound swab
Non-adherent sheet (optional)
Tubular bandage or crepe bandage (of appropriate size)
Adhesive tape
Disposal bag
Patient's prescription chart

Action	Rationale
Administer prescribed analgesia approximately 30 minutes prior to commencing the procedure.	To minimise pain and discomfort for the patient.
Assist the patient into a comfortable position with the neck well supported by pillows.	To allow ease of access to the ears and for the comfort of the patient.
Put on unsterile gloves and remove existing dressings, discard into the disposal bag.	To minimise the risk of cross infection.
Remove gloves and wash hands.	To minimise the risk of cross infection.
Assess the helix and anti-helix of the ear noting any oedema, redness, tenderness, pain and/or impaired hearing.	To detect early signs of complications e.g. chondritis (Purdue and Hunt, 1980) allowing for appropriate interventions to be performed (Sadowski, 1991).
If the ear appears red, inflamed and painful, take a bacteriological wound swab, label and send to the microbiology laboratory for culture and sensitivity.	To detect any infection which may delay healing or require treatment.
Apply sterile gloves and position the sterile towel across the patient's shoulders under the ears.	To prevent wetting or soiling of the patient's clothes or bed linen.
Moisten the sterile gauze with saline.	Moistened gauze will facilitate easier removal of old creams, exudate and/or crusts from the ear. Cotton wool should be avoided as the threads, if left *in situ* may provide a medium for the growth of organisms (Wood, 1976).
Gently but thoroughly clean the outer ear using each gauze swab once only.	To clean the ear and minimise the risk of cross infection.
Carefully remove all loose crusts from the outer ear but avoid removing any still firmly attached.	Removal of loose crusts helps to minimise the risk of infection. Removal of firmly attached crusts may cause further damage (Sadowski, 1991).
If any blisters are present, burst and expel the fluid but avoid removing any skin still firmly attached to the ear.	Deroofing blisters may cause excessive pain due to exposure of nerve endings. Removal of firmly attached skin may cause further damage.
Check the ear canal for the presence of old cream or exudate.	Removal helps to minimise infection.
Gently apply a large plug of paraffin gauze loosely into the outer ear canal.	To prevent the cream entering the external auditory canal (Orr and Hain, 1994).

Action	Rationale
Apply a layer of antibacterial cream (silver sulphadiazine) onto the burn areas on the outer ear, noting any exposed cartilage.	Exposed cartilage is at risk of infection (Kemble and Lamb, 1987; Settle 1986). Silver Sulphadiazine cream is a topical antibacterial agent indicated as an adjunct for the prevention and treatment of wound sepsis in patients with partial and full thickness burns (Hoffman, 1984).
Cover with 2–3 layers of paraffin gauze gently moulding it around the ear.	The use of paraffin gauze minimises dryness by maintaining a moist environment and prevents the dressing from adhering to the ear therefore minimising pain and discomfort for the patient on removal.
Apply gauze swabs behind the ear (between the ear and scalp).	Protects the cartilage and prevents contractures and/or webbing. The ear can become adhered to the head if adjacent burned surfaces are not separated (Sadowski, 1991).
Cover the paraffin gauze on the ear with layers of sterile gauze and Gamgee.	To absorb excess exudate and to provide a padded dressing for the comfort of the patient.
Secure the dressings in place with tubular bandage head dressing or a crepe bandage and secure with adhesive tape.	To prevent the dressings from becoming displaced. Tape is preferable to pins for the safety of the patient.
If tubular bandage or crepe bandage is unsuitable, continue as above but place a non-adherent sheet or pad under the patient's head across the pillows.	If the patient moves his or her head the non-stick sheet will prevent the ears from adhering to the pillows which can cause pain and further skin damage.
Remove gloves and sterile towel and wash hands.	
Assist the patient into a comfortable position ensuring no pressure from the dressings or pillows is applied to the ear. (A foam ring is a suitable alternative to pillows (Sadowski, 1991).	Pressure on the ears is painful and may cause impairment of blood circulation leading to necrosis. Avoiding pressure protects the cartilage from rubbing against the scalp.
Repeat the procedure daily or more frequently as required.	To minimise the risk of infection and to maintain a moist environment for healing to take place.
Record in the appropriate documentation.	To maintain an accurate record.

References

Dowling JA, Foley FD, Moncrief JA (1968) Chondritis in the burned ear. Plastic Reconstructive Surgery Volume 42, Number 2: 115.

Engrau LH (1987) Acute care and reconstruction of head and neck burns. In Boswick JA (ed.) The Art and Science of Burn Care. Rockville: MD — Aspen Publishers. p 336.

Goel TK, Law EJ, Macmillan BG (1983) Management of the acutely burned ear. Burns Journal 9: 218.

Hoffman S (1984) Silver sulphadiazine cream, an antibacterial agent for topical use in burns. A review of the literature. Scandinavian Journal of Plastic and Reconstructive Surgery 18: 18–19.

Kemble JVH, Lamb BE (1987) Practical Burns Management. London: Hodder and Stoughton.

Orr J, Hain T (1994) Burn wound management. An overview. Professional Nurse December: 153–6.

Purdue GF, Hunt JL (1980) Chronditis of the burned ear — A preventable complication. American Journal of Surgery 152: 257–9.

Sadowski DA (1991) Burns of the eyes and ears. In: Trofino RB (Ed) Nursing Care of the Burn-Injured Patient. Philadelphia: FA Davis Company. pp. 184–201.

Settle JAD (1986) Burns, the First Five Days. Hull: Smith and Nephew.

Wilson G, French G (1985) Plasticised polyvinylchloride as a temporary dressing for burns. British Medical Journal 294: 556–7.

Wood RAB (1976) Disintegration of cellulose dressing in open granulating wounds. British Medical Journal 785: 1444–5

Chapter 6
Care of a patient with burns to the face

Burns to the face are often a result of accidents involving explosions, e.g. flash burns, intense heat and/or flame burns or scalds.

In facial burns the eyes are usually protected by the closed eyelids. The involuntary blink reflex can be initiated by either tactile, visual or auditory stimuli (Guy et al., 1994). In most circumstances the normal pattern of injury is burn trauma to the eyelids with sparing around the crows foot and halo areas (Barnes, Mercer and Cochrane,1989).

Facial burns from flames will initially arouse suspicion of inhalation injuries hence the nurse will need to observe the patient closely on admission to the unit for the presence of soot in the mouth, singed nasal hairs and/or dry red mucous membranes to confirm this. It is important to report any abnormalities to the medical staff immediately.

Aspiration of hot fluids during scalding of the face may cause the development of laryngeal oedema and the nurse should closely monitor the patient's respiration rate. Deep burns of the face and burns to the tongue and pharynx may suggest the need for endotracheal intubation as the patient develops stridor and hoarseness. The extent of the burn injury and the position of the patient will influence the amount of oedema that will accumulate.

In the majority of cases the lax tissue of the face allows for enormous degrees of oedema. Within a few hours of the injury gross swelling of the eyelids and lips will occur which is maximal at 48 hours but which largely resolves in 4–5 days. Extensive psychological support will be required during this time not only for the patient but also for attending relatives and carers who may find the appearance very distressing. Positioning the patient in an upright position well supported by pillows will encourage drainage of oedema away from the face.

In the initial stages of a burn injury to the face it is difficult to estimate the depth of injury and early excision and skin grafting should be avoided.

1. Procedure for the care of a patient with burns to the face on admission to the Burns Unit

It is important that facial burns are assessed and treated by both medical and nursing staff who are adequately trained in burns care. Therefore admitting the patient to a Burns Unit is recommended.

Examination of burns to the face may provide detailed information on the type of burn injury, and prompt observations are required to determine the extent of injuries to the eyes, nose and mouth. Signs and symptoms may also indicate an inhalation injury and the patient may be at risk of developing respiratory distress only a few hours after injury.

See sections 1 and 2 in chapter 1 for advice on procedures.

Equipment

Clean tray/trolley
Sterile gloves
Fluorescein eye drops
Opthalmoscope or ultraviolet lamp
Sterile spatula
Patient's prescription chart
Nursing documentation charts
Light source (optional)

Action	Rationale
On admission to the Burns Unit, transfer the patient into a single room and nurse in protective isolation.	Protective isolation minimises the risk of cross infection to the patient which is likely if burns to the face are left exposed (Muir, Barclay and Settle, 1987).
Sit the patient in an upright position well supported by pillows.	To facilitate the drainage of oedema away from the face (Orr and Hain, 1994).
Obtain a detailed history of the injury, e.g. cause and duration of contact with the source.	To assist in ascertaining the severity of the injury. History allows for appropriate interventions to be performed (Sadowski, 1991).
Determine if any first aid treatment has been undertaken.	To assess whether the appropriate interventions have been performed.
Ask the patient if there is any pain, noting quality and intensity. Administer analgesia as prescribed by the medical staff.	To minimise pain and discomfort for the patient.
Perform a physical inspection:	
Observe the eyes for:	Observations assist with clinical assessment (Sadowski, 1991).
— Singed eyelashes and/or eyebrows. — Oedema of the eyelids and the inability to close the lids.	To indicate evidence of ocular damage (Sadowski, 1991).
— Opacity of the cornea. — Size, shape, equality of the pupils and the reaction to light.	Opacity may affect vision. Semi-dilated and/or fixed pupils signify an eye injury (Sadowski, 1991).

Action	Rationale
– Abrasions of the cornea and the presence of any foreign bodies.	
N.B. For a more detailed examination, the doctor may request the use of flourescein eye drops and an opthalmoscope or ultraviolet lamp.	Fluorescein temporarily stains the eye when examined through the opthalmoscope or using ultraviolet light and any damage to the cornea/conjunctiva will be evident.
Observe the nose for:	Observations assist with clinical assessment (Settle, 1986).
– Singed nasal hairs.	May indicate the patient has sustained an inhalation injury.
– Oedema of the nostrils.	May restrict nasal breathing.
– Abrasions, lacerations, bleeding.	
Observe the mouth for:	
– Soot (especially on the soft palate).	May indicate the patient has sustained an inhalation injury.
– Dry, red or damaged mucosa.	
– Burns or damage to the tongue.	
– Oedema of the lips, tongue, oropharynx and/or nasopharynx.	
N.B. For a more detailed examination, the doctor may request the use of a light source and a sterile spatula.	
Observe the face for:	
– Colour, e.g. blue, cherry red.	Bluish tinge may indicate cyanosis following an inhalation injury. Cherry red appearance may indicate inhalation of carbon monoxide (Bayley, 1991; Kinsella and Findlay, 1991).
– Abrasions, lacerations, bleeding.	
– Areas of skin loss and/or blisters.	To determine the percentage body surface area involved (Wilson, Fowler and Housden, 1987).
Record history and physical examination in the appropriate documentation.	To maintain an accurate record.

2. Procedure for the care of burns to the face

Facial care is aimed at patient comfort, promoting healing and minimising the risk of infection. Facial burns are normally nursed exposed in a clean, warm, dry, environment.

See sections 1–5 in Chapter 1 for advice on procedures

Equipment

Trolley
Sterile dressing pack
Sterile scissors
1 pair of sterile gloves
Sachet of normal saline and alcohol swab
Sterile gauze or sterile sponges
Sterile towel
Bacteriological wound swab (optional)
Soft paraffin or oily cream (optional)
Antibacterial cream (optional)
Hair clippers
Patient's prescription chart

Action	Rationale
Isolate the patient on admission in a single room until the face is dry.	Protective isolation minimises the risk of cross infection to the patient (Orr and Hain, 1994; Muir, Barclay and Settle, 1987).
Administer prescribed analgesia 30 minutes prior to commencing the procedure.	To minimise pain and discomfort for the patient during the procedure.
Sit the patient in an upright position well supported by pillows.	To facilitate the drainage of oedema away from the face (Orr and Hain, 1994).
Clip any facial hair as close to the skin as possible.	Hair may harbour micro-organisms that may cause infection in an open wound. Short facial hair allows for easier cleansing (Kemble and Lamb, 1987).
Avoid facial shaving until tolerated. The use of clippers is preferable until the face is completely healed.	To minimise pain and discomfort. As the beard grows, scabs may be lifted from the skin. Using clippers is an alternative method to shaving and for removing thick stubble.
Using the bacteriological wound swab gently wipe it over the face, label and send to the microbiology laboratory for culture and sensitivity.	To detect any infection which may delay healing or require treatment.
Apply sterile gloves and position the sterile towel across the patient's chest under the chin.	For the protection of the nurse and comfort of the patient.

Action	Rationale
Moisten the gauze swabs or sponges with saline and clean the face gently.	The use of cotton wool is avoided as it may leave fibres behind on the burn wound which may cause inflammation or infection (Wood, 1976). Regular cleansing minimises the risk of infection and minimises discomfort for the patient from serous fluid dripping into the ear, nose or mouth (Orr and Hain, 1994).
Using the sterile scissors, burst any blisters and expel the fluid that has collected beneath. Avoid deroofing the blisters.	Deroofing the blisters will cause pain by exposing nerve endings to the air.
Using the sterile scissors and forceps gently remove any loose scabs or dead tissue.	To remove any dead tissue that might harbour micro-organisms. To expose areas of re-epithelialisation.
Do not remove facial scabs before they have started to lift away from the skin.	To minimise the risk of facial scarring and to avoid damage to new epithelial cells (Settle, 1986).
Assess the burn and treat accordingly. For example: – Using sterile gauze/sponges apply saline soaks to the wet burn areas and then remove and leave the face exposed.	To minimise discomfort. To absorb wound exudate and minimise the risk of fluid dripping into the eyes, nose or ear of the patient (Orr and Hain, 1994). Exposure relieves distress from bulky facial dressings.
– Using sterile gauze/sponges apply a thin layer of silver sulphadiazine cream to the burn areas avoiding close contact with the eyes.	The surface of a partial thickness burn may be kept moist (not soggy) to encourage re-epithelialisation. Silver Sulphadiazine cream is an anti-bacterial cream effective in the treatment of burns (Hoffman, 1984) which minimises the risk of infection and helps to keep the wound moist to promote healing.
Repeat the above 4 steps, 2–4 hourly until the face stops exuding plasma.	To minimise the risk of infection and to maintain a moist wound environment to promote healing.
Position the patient upright well supported by pillows.	To facilitate drainage of oedema (Kemble and Lamb, 1987).
During the healing stage and when the face is dry, apply soft paraffin ointment or oily cream to any crusted areas.	To facilitate easy removal of dry crusts or scabs and to moisturise the new epithelium.

Action	Rationale
Perform daily wound assessments. (If skin grafting is required refer to appropriate procedure.)	To monitor and evaluate treatment.
Record in the appropriate documentation.	To maintain an accurate record.

References

Barnes SJ, Mercer DM, Cochrane TD (1989) Flash burns to the face. Journal of the International Society for Burn Injuries 15: 250–1.

Bayley EW (1991) Care of the burn patient with an inhalation injury. In: Trofino RB, (Ed) Nursing Care of the Burn-injured Patient Philadelphia: FA Davis p 331.

Guy PR, Taggart I, Adeniran A, Burd DA (1994) Corneal burns with eyelid sparing and their treatment. Journal of the International Society for Burn Injuries 20 (6): 561–3.

Hoffman S (1984) Silver sulphadiazine cream an anti-bacterial agent for topical use in burns. A Review of Literature. Scandinavian Journal of Plastic Reconstructive Surgery, 18: 18–19.

Kemble HJV, Lamb BE (1987) Burns of special sites. Practical Burns Management London: Hodder and Stoughton. p 177.

Kinsella J, Findlay J (1991) Carbon monoxide poisoning. Care of the Critically Ill. 7 (5): 182–4.

Muir IFK, Barclay TL, Settle JAD (1987) Burns and their Treatment 3rd edn, London: Butterworths. pp 63, 97.

Orr J, Hain T (1994) Burn wound management: An overview. Professional Nurse, December: 153–6.

Sadowski DA (1991) Burns of the eyes and ears. In: Trofino RB, (Ed) Nursing Care of the Burn-Injured Patient. Philadelphia: FA Davis. pp 184–201.

Settle JAD (1986) Burns: the First Five Days. Romford: Smith and Nephew Pharmaceuticals. pp 4–8.

Wilson GR, Fowler CA, Housden PL (1987) A new burn area assessment chart. Burns Journal 13 (5): 401–5.

Wood RAB (1976) Disintegration of cellulose dressings in open granulating wounds. British Medical Journal 785: 1444–5.

Chapter 7
Care of a patient with an inhalation injury

Inhalation injuries are amongst the most devastating types of trauma resulting from exposure to fire and smoke (Bayley, 1991). However, many of the patients who die from smoke inhalation injuries have no evidence of cutaneous burns.

Of all types of inhalation injury, carbon monoxide poisoning holds the greatest mortality rate and may be caused by faulty boilers, using gas engines in an enclosed space or inhaling car exhaust fumes either accidentally or as a suicide attempt (Bayley, 1991).

Upper airway obstruction

Direct heat may cause an injury to the structures of the upper respiratory tract and may also involve the oral cavity, pharynx, nasopharynx and/or vocal cords. As a result of the highly toxic gases, chemical burns may also occur (Bayley, 1991).

The patient will develop the following clinical signs:

1. Erythema and blistering of the oral and pharyngeal mucosa.
2. Laryngeal spasm.
3. Singed nasal hairs.
4. Sore throat/hoarseness.
5. Oedema — which causes obstruction of the airway.
6. Ulceration (in severe cases).

It is advised to consider securing the airway at an early stage in treatment rather than waiting until obvious clinical signs are evident. Control of the airway can be maintained by endotracheal intubation or tracheostomy (Clarke et al., 1990).

Lower airway damage

This usually occurs as a result of exposing the respiratory passages to chemicals (Bayley, 1991). Smoke from a fire is composed of liquid and solid particles in gases. The gases combine with water in the lungs to produce acids and alkalis that can be corrosive to the respiratory tract (Cioffi, Loring and Rue, 1991).

Following inhalation, movement of the cilia lining the respiratory tract ceases, therefore mucus and debris is not cleared. The inflammatory response causes oedema and congestion of the tracheobronchial tree as blood flow increases.

The patient may develop bronchospasm as a result of direct irritation of the airways and carbonaceous sputum may be expectorated in response to the chemical irritant.

The lining of the trachea and bronchi may become necrosed and may shed its epithelial lining.

Investigations

Numerous laboratory and diagnostic measures can help to make an early diagnosis of smoke inhalation and to assess the extent of damage. These include:

1. Arterial blood gas levels.
2. Carboxyhaemoglobin levels (Mather, 1986).
3. Fibreoptic bronchoscopy (Cioffi, Loring and Rue, 1991).
4. Chest X-ray.

Management

Management will depend on the severity of the injury and whether it is an upper or lower airway injury, but may include:

1. Tracheostomy.
2. Endotracheal tube.
3. Administration of 100% oxygen (Winter and Miller, 1976).
4. Administration of humidified oxygen.
5. Administration of intravenous bronchodilators.
6. Nebulisers.
7. Physiotherapy, e.g. postural drainage, coughing and deep breathing exercises.
8. Mechanical ventilation.

If patients survive the critical phase following a severe inhalation burn injury they may still be at risk of developing complications, e.g. pulmonary oedema, bronchopneumonia, persistent cough due to airway irritation, chronic bronchitis and/or tracheal stenosis.

1. Procedure for the care of a patient with an inhalation injury on admission to the Burns Unit

All patients who have sustained an inhalation injury will require close monitoring of the airway and their breathing and will require numerous laboratory and other diagnostic measures to assist not only in making an early diagnosis of smoke inhalation but also in assessing the extent of the damage. Admission to hospital is advisable for all patients who have inhaled smoke or have a history suggestive of a respiratory burn.

See sections 1 and 2 in Chapter 1 for advice on procedures.

Equipment

Trolley
Oxygen supply
Flow meter
Oxygen tubing
Humidifier and sterile water
Mask or nasal cannulae
Unsterile gloves
Burns assessment chart
Nursing documentation charts

Action	Rationale
On admission of the patient to the Burns Unit secure and maintain a clear airway.	The heat of a burn may cause upper airway obstruction and result in respiratory complications (Wilding, 1990).
Sit the patient upright well supported by pillows.	Sitting upright assists the patient with breathing (Wilding, 1990).
Remove any jewellery from around the neck.	If any swelling is present around the neck a tightly fitting necklace may constrict the airway and interfere with respiration.
Obtain a detailed history of the injury to include: – Type of burning material	To assist in ascertaining the severity of the injury. History allows for appropriate interventions to be performed (Coiffi, Loring and Rue, 1991; Wilding, 1990).
– Length of time the patient was in contact with the source. – A description of the physical environment of the accident, e.g. enclosed, well ventilated, out of doors etc.	To assist in ascertaining the severity of the injury.
– Condition of the patient when rescued, history of loss of consciousness.	To assist in ascertaining the severity of the injury.
Apply unsterile gloves.	For the protection of the nurse against body fluids.
Perform a physical inspection of the face and neck. Observe:	Swelling of the face and/or neck leads to direct obstruction of the upper airway.

Action	Rationale
– Evidence of any oedema on the face/neck. – Extent of any skin loss on the face/neck.	To determine the percentage body surface area of the burn (Wilson, Fowler and Housden, 1987).
– Evidence of cyanosis or cherry red appearance.	Cyanosis indicates poor oxygenation. A cherry red appearance indicates carbon monoxide poisoning (Kinsella and Findlay, 1991).
– Singed eyelashes/eyebrows.	Loss of eyelashes/eyebrows may indicate an explosion at the scene of the accident and the possibility of direct thermal injuries to the airways.
– Presence of soot in the nostrils and/or singed nasal hairs.	Presence confirms upper airway injury.
– Presence of soot in the mouth, damaged oral mucosa.	Respiratory manifestations develop in response to smoke inhalation (Bayley, 1991). Their presence confirms an inhalation injury.
– Circumferential or full thickness burns to the neck.	Circumferential and/or full thickness burns may cause constriction of the airway and respiratory distress.
N.B. Escharotomy may be required for circumferential burns of the neck/trunk (See Chapter 8 for the procedure for Escharotomy).	Escharotomy allows for expansion of skin to accommodate swelling (Konop, 1991) and to minimise tracheal obstruction and to free respiratory movements.
Observe for evidence of stridor, dyspnoea, wheezing and/or hoarseness of voice.	Respiratory manifestations development in response to smoke inhalation (Bayley, 1991). Observations may detect signs and symptoms of airway dysfunction.
Record type, depth and rate of respirations.	To detect signs and symptoms of airway dysfunction.
Record the history and physical examination in the appropriate documentation.	To maintain an accurate record.
Administer humidified oxygen therapy as prescribed via mask or nasal cannulae.	To promote oxygenation and prevent hypoxaemia To maintain oxygen levels over 10 kPa (Wilding, 1990).

2. Procedure for the care of a patient with carbon monoxide poisoning on admission to the Burns Unit

Introduction

Carbon monoxide is a colourless, odourless gas produced by the incomplete combustion of carbon-containing compounds (Kinsella and Findlay, 1991). Sources of carbon monoxide poisoning are car exhaust fumes, fires, and poorly ventilated or defective heating appliances.

Carbon monoxide combines strongly with haemoglobin causing impairment of oxygen transport. In addition there is evidence of direct tissue toxicity. Carbon monoxide poisoning presents clinical signs and symptoms ranging from nausea and headache, to coma and convulsions, therefore, early active treatment is required.

Immediate treatment of carbon monoxide poisoning is with high concentrations of oxygen. However, giving hyperbaric oxygen is also recommended (Broome, Pearson and Skrine, 1988; Anon, 1988) to patients who are, or who have been unconscious, pregnant women, patients with neurological and/or cardiac complications and those patients with carboxyhaemoglobin concentrations greater than 40%.

See sections 1 and 2 in Chapter 1 for advice on procedures

Equipment

Trolley
Oxygen supply
Flow meter
Oxygen tubing
Ventimask or oronasal mask
Blood gas flow chart
Nursing documentation charts
ECG monitor and leads
Observation charts
Ophthalmoscope or small torch
Patient's treatment card

Action	Rationale
On admission of the patient to the Burns Unit secure and maintain a clear airway.	To minimise the risk of respiratory complications.
Sit the patient upright well supported by pillows.	Sitting upright assists the patient with breathing (Wilding, 1990).
Obtain a detailed history of the injury.	To assist in ascertaining the severity of the injury. History allows for appropriate interventions to be performed (Coiffi and Rue, 1991; Wilding, 1990).

Action	Rationale
Observe the patient for impaired levels of consciousness.	Altered consciousness levels may indicate cerebral anoxia (Langford and Armstrong, 1989).
Administer a high concentration and a high flow of oxygen to the patient using a high airflow mask with oxygen enrichment such as the Ventimask, or a tight fitting oronasal mask connected to a breathing system.	To avoid immediate and long-term cerebral damage caused by carbon monoxide poisoning (Myers, Synder and Enhoff, 1985). Some of the commercially available masks achieve variable and unpredictable oxygen concentrations that depend on the patient's respiratory rate, tidal volume and rate of inspiratory air flow (Langford and Armstrong, 1989). Ventimask can achieve 60% inspired concentration (Campbell, 1982).
Assist the doctor in obtaining a sample of arterial blood from the femoral, brachial or radial artery for blood gas analysis and measurement of carboxyhaemoglobin.	Blood gas investigation is the measurement of the tension of oxygen and carbon dioxide in arterial blood and may be used to detect carboxyhaemoglobin poisoning (Carrougher and Gretchen, 1993). The blood level of carboxyhaemoglobin may also relate to the symptomatology.
N.B. If repeated samples are recommended it may be advisable to site an arterial line.	For the comfort of the patient, to avoid repeated needle sticks and to provide easy access to arterial blood.
Observe the patient for:	
– Headache.	Cerebral hypoxia leads to a throbbing headache due to cerebral vasodilation (Kinsella and Findlay, 1991).
– Ventricular arrhythmias, ECG changes of ischaemia and myocardial infarction.	In the cardiovascular system myocardial ischaemia and dysfunction occur even in the normal heart at high levels of carbon monoxide and in diseased hearts at lower levels (Kinsella and Findlay, 1991; Walden and Gottlieb, 1990).
– Neurological symptoms e.g. extrapyramidal rigidity, papilloedema and flame-shaped haemorrhages in the eye.	Evidence of neurological symptoms indicates carbon monoxide poisoning.
– Colour.	Patients who have sustained carbon monoxide poisoning may have a cherry red appearance (Bayley, 1991; Kinsella and Findlay, 1991).
– Confusion, disorientation and/or loss of consciousness.	The presence of confusion, disorientation and/or loss of consciousness indicates hypoxia (Langford and Armstrong, 1989).

Action	Rationale
Commence a blood gas flow chart and record levels of carboxyhaemoglobin and report any changes to medical staff immediately.	In acute carbon monoxide poisoning symptoms may be manifested according to the level of carboxyhaemoglobin. Levels between 10% and 30% are charaterised by headache, confusion and exertional dyspnoea. At around 40% unconsciousness may occur (Kinsella and Findlay, 1991) and at levels in excess of 60% convulsions and death may occur (Meredith and Vale, 1988).
Continue to monitor and record airway and breathing.	To detect early signs of complications and respiratory distress.
Refer the patient to the medical staff and the Intensive Care Unit if respiratory distress progresses.	The patient may require intubation and intermittent positive pressure ventilation (Langford and Armstrong, 1989).
Record progress on the appropriate chart and in the nursing documentation.	To maintain an accurate record.
In extreme cases the patient may need to be transferred to a hyperbaric oxygen chamber for further treatment.	Hyperbaric oxygen increases the amount of oxygen dissolved in plasma, improving oxygen delivery to the tissues (Broome, Pearson and Skrine, 1988; Anon, 1988). This also combats the directly toxic effects of carbon monoxide in tissues (Langford and Armstrong, 1989).
Thereafter, administer oxygen therapy as prescribed by the medical staff in accordance with the blood gas levels.	To maintain normal levels of oxygen saturation in the blood and delivery to the tissues.

3. Procedure for the care of a patient with an inhalation injury

Following extensive burn injuries the respiratory system is subject to a wide variety of insults. Damage may have occurred via direct thermal injuries to the upper airways from breathing in flames or hot gases, or from chemical damage to the lower airway as a consequence of inhaling smoke containing corrosive and/or toxic products of combustion (Settle, 1986).

See sections 1, 2 and 5 in Chapter 1 for advice on procedures and sharps policy.

Equipment

Trolley
Oxygen supply
Flow meter
Oxygen tubing

Humidifier and sterile water
Mask or nasal cannulae
Unsterile gloves
Sterile tracheostomy pack (optional)
Sputum pot and tissues
Universal specimen container
Pulse oximeter machine and appropriate probe
Cardboard tray/receiver
Alcohol wipe
Heparinised 2 ml syringe and needle
Nebuliser and prescribed bronchodilator solution
Patient's prescription card
Mouth wash solution or lemon and glycerine swabs
Nursing documentation
Appropriate flow charts
Sharps box

Action	Rationale
Sit the patient upright well supported by pillows.	Sitting upright allows for full chest expansion and assists with breathing (Wilding, 1990).
Administer humidified oxygen as prescribed via mask or nasal cannulae.	Oxygen therapy will deliver more oxygen to the tissues in a state of hypoxia. Humidified oxygen increases the moisture content of inspired gases and assists the function of the upper airway (Wilding, 1990).
Offer mouth care frequently.	To prevent a dry sore mouth.
Observe for evidence of stridor, dyspnoea, wheezing and bronchospasm.	Evidence will indicate airway dysfunction. Impending respiratory obstruction or effects of carbon monoxide poisoning (Bayley, 1991).
If bronchospasm is present administer bronchodilators as prescribed on the patient's prescription chart using a nebuliser.	To decrease bronchospasm by relaxing the bronchial muscles and dilating the airway (Chu, 1981).
Record type, depth and rate of respirations.	To detect change in airway dysfunction and to evaluate the progression of respiratory effects of smoke inhalation (Carrougher and Gretchen, 1993).
Ensure the patient is given a sputum pot and tissues.	For the comfort of the patient and to allow for inspection of any pulmonary secretions.
Observe and record amount, colour and consistency of any pulmonary secretions.	Carbonaceous sputum may indicate lower airway injury. The presence of infection will cause changes in the colour, consistency and amount of sputum.

Action	Rationale
Obtain a sputum specimen (if required) in a universal specimen container. Label and send to the microbiology laboratory for culture and sensitivity.	To detect any signs of bacterial infection.
If expectoration is difficult, refer the patient to a physiotherapist and assist with postural drainage (if required).	To improve the pattern of breathing and to assist coughing which helps to clear the major bronchi of secretions.
Assist with positioning the patient for an X-ray (if required).	An X-ray provides an indication of the progression of the effects of the inhalation injury and response to treatment (Coiffi, Loring and Rue, 1991).
Assist the doctor in obtaining a sample of arterial blood from the femoral, bronchial or radial artery.	Blood gas investigation is the measurement of the tension of oxygen and carbon dioxide in arterial blood. It provides an indication of the development of respiratory acidosis and tissue hypoxaemia and may be used to detect carboxyhaemoglobin poisoning (Carrougher and Gretchen, 1993).
Record the patient's temperature, the current percentage of oxygen being delivered and the present haemoglobin level (if known) and send this information with the sample to the laboratory.	The blood gas analyser calibrates the results of the sample according to these variables.
Commence a blood gas flow chart, if repeated arterial blood gas samples are required.	To monitor serial arterial blood gases. Inadequate ventilation results in decreased oxygen and increased carbon dioxide levels over time.
N.B. If repeat samples are recommended it may be advisable to site an arterial line.	For the comfort of the patient, to avoid repeated needle sticks and to provide easy access to arterial blood.
Prepare the pulse oximeter machine: – Attach a probe to the finger, toe or ear lobe. – Switch on the machine. – Observe and record the result.	To allow for close monitoring of the oxygen saturation levels. Normal range is between 98% and 100% (Carrougher and Gretchen, 1993).
Observe the patient for any signs of confusion, disorientation and/or loss of consciousness.	The presence of confusion, disorientation and/or loss of consciousness indicates hypoxia (Langford and Armstrong, 1989).

Action	Rationale
Continue to monitor and record airway and breathing half to 1 hourly as requested by the medical staff and report any negative changes immediately.	To detect early signs of complications and respiratory distress.
Monitor intake and output — avoid fluid overload.	Monitoring fluid balance minimises the risk of pulmonary oedema which decreases the ability of oxygen and carbon dioxide to exchange at alveolar level (Bayley, 1991).
Refer the patient to the medical staff and the Intensive Care Unit if respiratory distress progresses.	The patient may require ventilatory support to assist with breathing (Venus, 1987).
Provide adequate rest.	Rest decreases metabolic rate and oxygen consumption by muscles, thereby allowing more oxygen to be available for vital organ function (Bayley, 1991).
Record progress on the appropriate chart and in the nursing documentation.	To maintain an accurate record.

4. Procedure for care of the mouth

Burn trauma patients need regular effective mouth care because:

1. They may be nil by mouth following major burn trauma injuries due to the risk of paralytic ileus.
2. An inhalation injury may damage the oral mucosa.
3. They may be unable to care for their own oral hygiene.
4. Some drugs affect the oral mucosa, e.g. antibiotics disturb normal flora.
5. Dehydration prevents salivary glands from functioning normally.
6. Poor nutrition affects the health of the oral mucosa.
7. Plaque and debris form on teeth, irrespective of whether or not the patient is able to eat and drink.

Mouth care should be planned daily and be based on individual patient assessment (Jenkins, 1989). Plaque causes dental cavities and peridontal disease if it is not removed and patients are at risk of developing dental decay and gum disease (Clarke, 1993).

See sections 1 and 2 in Chapter 1 for advice on procedures.

Equipment

Soft toothbrush with a small head
Toothpaste with fluoride

Mouth care pack
Mouthwash solution
Soft paraffin
1 pair of unsterile gloves
Water
20 ml syringe and quill
Yankhauer suction catheter
Suction apparatus
Patient's prescription chart
Torch (optional)
Tongue depressor (optional)

Action	Rationale
Assess the condition of the patient's mouth and teeth using a torch, tongue depressor or gloved finger.	To determine risk factors that may make the patient susceptible to oral problems, e.g. dryness, colour, texture, presence of plaque debris, lesions, bleeding (Clarke, 1993). To decide on an appropriate method of oral care (De Walt 1975; Harrison, 1987).
Apply unsterile gloves.	To minimise the risk of cross infection to both the patient and nurse (Shepherd, Page and Sammon, 1987).
Using a soft toothbrush and a small amount of toothpaste, brush around the teeth and gums.	To remove plaque and debris and to freshen the mouth (Gooch, 1985). The toothbrush is an ideal tool for removing bacterial plaque (Nelsley, 1986; Watson, 1989). Cleaning with foam sticks or gauze is ineffective (Liwu, 1989).
Rinse with water (using syringe and continuous low suction if the patient is unable to rinse own mouth).	To remove residual toothpaste (Gooch, 1985). If toothpaste is not rinsed away properly it has a drying effect on the oral mucosa (Gooch, 1985).
Every 2–3 hours rinse the mouth with mouthwash solution and water.	To maintain oral hygiene and reduce the risk of changes to the oral mucosa (De Walt and Haines, 1969). The mouth should be kept moist, as dry tissue is subject to infection and decreased salivary flow facilitates plaque accumulation (Block, 1976).
If the mouth is sore or ulcerated, do not use a toothbrush or hydrogen peroxide. Rinse gently with a diluted mouthwash solution.	To maintain oral hygiene whilst minimising further pain or discomfort (Shepherd, Page and Sammon, 1987).

Action	Rationale
Observe the mouth for evidence of infection, e.g. thrush and administer prescribed medication, e.g. Nystatin suspension.	To treat the infection (Nelsley, 1986). Oral candidiasis (thrush) is a common fungal infection and presents as white spots in the mouth. Nystatin suspension is an effective treatment (Clarke, 1993).
Following oral care apply a light coating of soft paraffin to the lips.	To prevent dehydration of the lips (Gibbons, 1983). Soft paraffin appears to be effective in preventing the lips from becoming dry, cracked and sore (Maurer, 1977; McCord and Stalker, 1988).
Dispose of mouth care pack and mouthwash solution every 24 hours.	To minimise the risk of cross infection.
Rinse and dry toothbrush.	To minimise the risk of cross infection.
Repeat the procedure 3 times daily or more often as required.	For the comfort of the patient and to minimise the risk of oral infections developing.
If the patient has dentures these should be cleaned daily using cold water, a soft toothbrush and washing-up detergent. If not being worn, soak in water or a denture cleaning agent and change the water daily.	Toothpaste and scouring powders can damage the denture surface (Clarke, 1993). Hot water will warp dentures as will leaving them dry (McCord and Stalker, 1988).

References

Anon (1988) Treatment of carbon monoxide poisoning. Drug and Therapeutic Bulletin 26 (20): 77–9.

Bayley EW (1991) Care of the burn patient with an inhalation injury. In: Trofino RB, (Ed) Management of the Burn-Injured Patient. Philadelphia: FA Davis. pp 325–47.

Block PL (1976) Dental health in hospitalised patients. American Journal of Nursing. 76: 1162–4.

Broome JR, Pearson RR, Skrine H (1988) Carbon monoxide poisoning. Forgotten not gone. British Journal of Hospital Medicine 39: 298–305.

Campbell EJM (1982) How to use the Venturimask. Lancet II: 1206.

Carroughter GJ, Gretchen J (1993) Inhalation injury. American Association of Clinical Nursing — Clinical Issues 4 (2): 367–76.

Chu C (1981) New concepts of pulmonary burn injury. Journal of Trauma 21: 958–61.

Cioffi WG, Loring W, Rue I (1991) Diagnosis and treatment of inhalation injuries. Critical Care Clinics of North America 3 (2): 191–8.

Cioffi WG, Rue LW (1991) Diagnosis and treatment of inhalation injuries. Critical Care Clinics of North America 3: 191–8.

Clarke G (1993) Mouth care and the hospitalised patient. British Journal of Nursing. 2 (4): 225–7.

Clarke WR, Bonaventura M, Myers W, Kellman R (1990) Smoke inhalation and airway management at a regional burns unit 1974–1983. Part II — Airway management. Journal of Burn Care and Rehabilitation II: 121.

De Walt E (1975) Effect of timed hygiene measures on oral mucosa in a group of elderly subjects. Nursing Research 24: 104–8.

De Walt, Haines AK (1969) The effects of specified stressors on healthy mucosa. Nursing Research 18 (1): 22–7.

Gibbons DE (1983) Mouth care procedures. Nursing Times 79 (7): 30.

Gooch J (1985) Mouth care. Professional Nurse 1 (3): 77–8.

Harrison A (1987) Oral hygiene, denture care. Nursing Times Volume 83 (19): 28–9.

Jenkins DA (1989) Oral care in ICU. An important nursing role. Nursing Standard. 8 (4): 24–8.

Kinsella J, Findlay J (1991) Carbon monoxide poisoning. Care of the Critically Ill 7 (5): 182–4.

Konop DJ (1991) General local treatment. In: Trofino RB, (Ed) Management of the Burn-Injured Patient. Philadelphia: FA Davis. pp 55–6.

Langford RM, Armstrong RF (1989) Algorithm for managing injury from smoke inhalation. British Medical Journal 200: 902–5.

Liwu A (1989) Oral hygiene in intubated patients. Australian Journal of Advanced Nursing. 7 (2): 47.

Mather J (1986) Inhalation injury in major burns. Care of the Critically Ill 2 (5): 17.

Maurer J (1977) Providing optimal oral health. Nursing Clinics of North America. 2 (4): 671–5.

McCord F, Stalker A (1988) Brushing up on oral care. Nursing Times. 84 (13): 40–1.

Meredith T, Vale A (1988) Carbon monoxide poisoning. British Medical Journal 296: 77–9.

Myers RAM, Synder SK, Enhoff TA (1985) Sub-acute sequelae of carbon monoxide poisoning. Annals of Emergency Medicine 14 (1): 1163–7.

Nelsley L (1986) Mouth care and the intubated patient — The aim of preventing infections. Intensive Care Nursing 1(4): 187–93.

Settle JAD (1986) Burns the First Five Days. Romford: Smith and Nephew. Essex.

Shepherd G, Page C, Sammon P (1987) Oral hygiene the mouth trap. Nursing Times 83 (19): 23–7.

Venus B (1987) Prophylactic intubation and continuous positive airway pressure in the management of inhalation injury in burn victims. Critical Care Medicine 9: 519.

Walden SM, Gottlieb SO (1990) Urban angina, urban arrythmias — carbon monoxide and the heart. Annals of International Medicine 113: 337–8.

Watson R (1989) Care of the mouth. Nursing. 3 (44): 20–4.

Wilding PA (1990) Care of respiratory burns — hard work can bring spectacular results. Professional Nurse, May: 412–9.

Wilson GR, Fowler CA, Housden PL (1987) A new burn area assessment chart. Burns Journal 13 (5): 401–5.

Winter FM, Miller JN (1976) Carbon monoxide poisoning. Journal of American Medical Association 236: 502.

Further Reading

Barnett J (1991) A reassessment of oral health care. Professional Nurse 6 (12): 703–8.

Kemble JVH, Lamb B (1987) Practical Burns Management. London: Hodder and Stoughton. pp 125–43.

Millinson K (1991) Taking care of John's mouth. Nursing Times 87 (21): 34–5.

Thompson PB (1986) Effect on mortality of inhalation injury. Journal of Trauma 26: 163.

Torrance C (1990) Oral hygiene. Surgical Nurse 3 (4): 16–20.

Chapter 8
Care of a patient with circumferential burns

Following a burn injury, the capillaries become more permeable, fluid moves from the intravascular to the extravascular space and generalised oedema accumulates in and around the burn wound (Konop, 1991).

In normal circumstances the skin is soft, supple and elastic. However, in a patient who has sustained full thickness burns the skin becomes hard, leathery and inelastic. When this is coupled with a circumferential burn around the neck, chest or limb, the effects could result in loss of life or limb.

Circumferential full thickness burns cause a tourniquet effect as the skin is unable to stretch sufficiently to accommodate the increasing swelling caused by the oedema (Konop, 1991).

In patients who have burns to the neck or chest the trachea may be constricted and expansion of the lungs may be restricted causing respiratory complications. In cases of circumferential burns to a limb or extremity the tourniquet effect hinders arterial flow and increases venous congestion, therefore impeding circulation.

Treatment for these cases is to perform an escharotomy. Konop (1991) defines an escharotomy as a linear incision extending through the burn eschar down to superficial fat. It allows the skin to expand in order to accommodate the swelling and to permit unrestricted blood flow to the distal area of the extremity. The procedure can only be performed by a doctor.

Indications for escharotomy

1. Increase in size and tightness of the burn area.
2. Respiratory embarrassment due to burns to the neck/chest
3. If burns to a limb/extremity result in:

   absent or diminishing pulses
   pain, tingling sensation, numbness
   slow capillary refill
   cool to the touch.
   distal cyanosis/pallor

Siting of escharotomies

The doctor performing the procedure must take into consideration the scarring that will occur as a result. Correct siting is important both to relieve the tension and to provide a scar that can easily be concealed. See Figure 8.1.

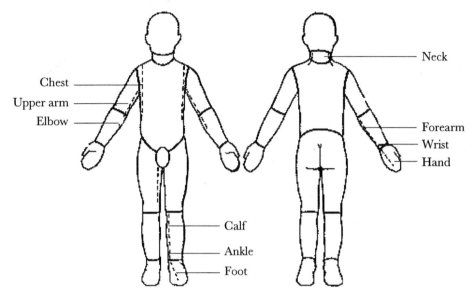

Figure 8.1 *The siting of escharotomies.*

Sites include:

1. Chest — vertical incision lateral to the nipple or a chequer-board effect.
2. Neck — vertical incision laterally to both sides.
3. Upper arm/elbow — along the medial aspect.
4. Forearm/wrist — along the medial aspect
5. Hand — axially on the dorsum.
6. Fingers — midlateral incision.
7. Abdomen — vertically in both loins.
8. Calf/Ankle — along the medial aspect.
9. Foot — on the dorsum. (Kemble and Lamb 1987)

Complications of escharotomy

The patient may experience pain and anxiety. In a full thickness burn, nerve endings are destroyed. Sedation or analgesia may be prescribed to minimise anxiety and any discomfort that may be experienced during and after the procedure.

Bleeding may occur with an escharotomy procedure but can usually be controlled with manual pressure, pressure dressings or the use of alginate wound care products.

Antibacterial agents may be applied topically as part of the wound care to minimise infection.

1. Procedure for an escharotomy

An escharotomy is a linear incision extending through the burn eschar down to superficial fat (Konop, 1991). It is only performed by a member of the medical staff. However, a nurse will be required to assist throughout.

See sections 1 - 5 in Chapter 1 for advice on procedures and sharps policy.

Equipment

Trolley
Sterile dressing pack
2 pairs of sterile gloves
Sterile scalpel (or sterile blade and handle)
Sterile linen towel/Goretex sheet
Alginate wound product (of choice)
Paraffin gauze
Antibacterial cream (Silver Sulphadiazine — optional)
Skin antiseptic solution (10% Povidone Iodine with alcohol or alcoholic Chlorhexidine 0.5% — red)
Sterile gauze swabs
Gamgee
Crepe bandage (of appropriate size)
Adhesive tape
Extra pair of sterile and unsterile gloves (if required)
Sharps box
Patient's prescription chart

Action	Rationale
Administer analgesia or sedation as prescribed on the patient's prescription chart, 15–30 minutes prior to commencing the procedure.	In a full thickness burn nerve endings are destroyed and the procedure should be painless (Settle, 1986) but it may still cause some anxiety and discomfort for the patient. Administration of analgesia or sedation should minimise anxiety and discomfort (Konop, 1991).
The nurse:	
– Apply sterile gloves.	To maintain asepsis.
– Place the limb on the sterile towel/Goretex sheet.	To minimise the risk of infection and maintain asepsis.
The doctor:	
– Open the sterile pack. – Apply sterile gloves. – Moisten the gauze swabs with the antiseptic solution of choice.	To maintain asepsis.

Action	Rationale
– Clean the skin.	To minimise the risk of infection.
– Using the scalpel, make a medial and/or lateral incision along the length of the circumferential burn.	To allow for the expansion of the skin caused by the development of oedema and to allow unrestricted blood flow to the distal end of the extremity (Konop, 1991).
– Escharotomies to the chest may be performed using multiple incisions to produce a chequer-board effect.	To allow for maximum chest expansion and achievement of adequate respiration (Settle, 1986).
– Using a gauze swab apply firm pressure to any bleeding points for 2–5 minutes.	Bleeding is a natural occurrence during the procedure. Applying pressure may control any bleeding points (Konop, 1991).
Redress the wounds according to the doctor's instructions:	
– Apply an alginate product directly to the wound or loosely pack the incisions with alginate rope or ribbon.	Alginates are useful agents in treating bleeding wounds as they have anticoagulant properties (Groves and Lawrence, 1986).
or	
– Apply a thin layer of Silver Sulphadiazine cream and cover with 2–3 layers of paraffin gauze directly to the wound.	Silver Sulphadiazine cream is an antibacterial agent which minimises infection (Hoffman, 1984; Hamilton-Miller, Shah and Smith, 1993). Paraffin gauze is a bleached cotton gauze impregnated with soft paraffin and is ideal as a non-stick dressing (Thomas, 1994).
– Cover with several layers of sterile gauze and Gamgee.	To absorb any bleeding that may occur.
– Firmly apply bandage(s) of appropriate size and secure with adhesive tape.	Firm bandaging assists with applying pressure to control bleeding.
or	
– If escharotomies have been performed to fingers or toes, apply a layer of Silver Sulphadiazine cream to the wounds or apply an alginate dressing to the incision sites and cover with a plastic bag secured at the wrist or ankle with gauze and a bandage.	Silver Sulphadiazine cream is an antibacterial agent and minimises the risk of infection (Hoffman, 1984; Hamilton-Miller, Shah and Smith, 1993). The use of a plastic bag facilitates easier visual and sensory observations of the extremity. Alginates are useful agents in treating bleeding wounds as they have anticoagulant properties (Groves and Lawrence, 1986)
Remove gloves and wash hands.	
Elevate limb appropriately:	To relieve venous congestion and to minimise oedema collecting in the affected limb (Sykes and Bailey, 1975).
– Legs on pillows.	
– Arms in slings (above the level of the heart).	
– Chest — sit the patient upright, well supported by pillows.	To assist the patient with breathing.

Action	Rationale
Increase the temperature of the environment.	If the patient is cold, peripheral vessels constrict impeding blood flow (Childs, 1994).
Continue to monitor and record the circulation of the extremities half to 1 hourly noting strength of pulse, warmth and colour of the skin, capillary refill and sensation.	If the extremity becomes cool, cyanosed/blanched has a weak pulse, slow capillary refill and reduced sensation, further escharotomies may be necessary.
If the chest is involved, monitor and record the respiration rate, difficulty in breathing and evidence of cyanosis, half to 1 hourly.	If the patient is experiencing difficulty in breathing further escharotomies may be necessary.
If the dressings become wet or blood stained:	
– Apply unsterile gloves.	To protect the nurse from body fluids.
– Remove the outer bandage and any wet dressings underneath. **Do not** remove any dressings that are stuck.	To minimise the risk of cross infection, (as wet dressings encourage the growth of micro-organisms) and for the comfort of the patient. Removing adherent dressings may cause further bleeding to occur.
– Discard dressings in disposal bag, remove gloves and wash hands.	
– Observe the amount of bleeding. If excessive inform the medical staff and remove all dressings.	If the bleeding is excessive the patient may require further investigations of the wound as a blood vessel may be severed and require tying off.
– Apply sterile gloves.	To maintain asepsis.
– Redress the wound using an alginate product or paraffin gauze (as appropriate). Cover with sterile gauze, Gamgee and crepe bandage. Secure with adhesive tape.	Alginates are useful agents in treating bleeding wounds (Groves and Lawrence, 1986). Paraffin gauze is an ideal non-adherent dressing (Thomas, 1994), gauze and Gamgee is used to absorb any further leakage. Tape is preferable to pins for the safety of the patient.
– Remove gloves and wash hands.	
Ensure the patient is left as comfortable as possible and administer analgesia as prescribed on a regular basis.	To minimise pain and discomfort for the patient.
Record in the appropriate documentation.	To maintain an accurate record.

References

Childs C (1994) Temperature regulation in burned patients. British Journal of Intensive Care. April: 129–34.

Groves AR, Lawrence JC (1986) Alginate dressings as donor site thermostat. Annals of Royal College of Surgeons of England 68: 27.

Hamilton-Miller JMT, Shah S, Smith C (1993) Silver sulphadiasine. A comprehensive *in vitro* reassessment. Chemotherapy 39: 405–9.

Hoffman S (1984) Silver sulphadiasine cream an antibacterial agent for topical use in burns. A review of the literature. Scandinavian Journal of Plastic and Reconstructive Surgery 18: 18–19.

Kemble HJV, Lamb BE (1987) Practical Burns Management. London: Hodder and Stoughton. pp 36–7.

Konop DJ (1991) General local treatment. In: Trofino RB, (Ed) Nursing Care of the Burn-Injured Patient, Philadelphia: FA Davies. pp 55–6.

Settle JAD (1986) Burns the First Five Days. Romford: Smith and Nephew.

Sykes PJ, Bailey BN (1975) Treatment of hand burns with occlusive bags. A comparison of three methods. Burns Journal 2: 163.

Thomas S (1994) Jelonet. In: Thomas S, (Ed) Handbook of Wound Dressings. London: MacMillan. pp 108–9.

Further Reading

Morgan B, Wright M (1986) Essentials of plastic and reconstructive surgery. London: Faber and Faber.

Chapter 9
Care of patient with burns to the hand

Burns to the hands may occur as a result of electricity, frostbite, chemicals or flames. Hands are common sites for current entry and exit wounds in electrical burns, and on physical examination local tissue destruction is less than the damage that may have occurred to other body organs (Martin, 1991). The wound may appear dry and charred and involve cutaneous and subcutaneous tissue and in many cases will require surgical excision and skin grafting.

The hands are also vulnerable areas to frostbite. They will appear pale and waxy with some localised oedema and poor circulation. Recommended treatment is to immerse the affected part in water at 38.7–40.6° C (Martin, 1991) in order to re-warm it. Over-exposure of the hand to heat sources or continually rubbing the area should be avoided as it may cause further damage.

With burns following chemical injuries tissue damage may continue for up to 72 hours post injury if adequate first aid treatment is not performed. Continuous irrigation of the skin with water (in the initial stages) to dilute the chemical is very important and may be continued following admission to hospital. The wound may appear superficial but can progress to full thickness.

In adults, flame burns to the hands often occur as a result of attempts to beat out flames that may be engulfing the individual or another victim (Kemble and Lamb, 1984). As the skin on the palmer surface is thicker in comparison to the dorsal surface, the burn is usually full thickness on the dorsum and may expose joints and extensor tendons.

One of the priorities in caring for burns to the hands is to promote lymphatic and venous drainage by elevating the limb to minimise oedema. Frequent and regular muscle movement of the hand(s) should be encouraged to minimise joint stiffness and preserve function (Muddiman, 1989). Other aims of treatment include minimising the risk of infection to the wound surface and providing an environment beneficial to wound healing.

When burns to the hand are circumferential and/or involve the fingers it is recommended that a plastic or Goretex bag should be applied as opposed to bulky finger dressings, to allow for active exercises to be performed without the restriction of bandages.

In patients who are unable to move the hands adequately or who are at risk of developing contractures, individualised splints may be applied to minimise the risk of stiff, non-functional positions of the hand. These are applied over the bag or dressings, secured with velcro or bandage and are regularly assessed by the physiotherapist usually on a daily basis.

With full thickness burns to the hands, early excision and skin grafting within 3–4 days post injury is advised, to enable early mobilisation and minimise joint stiffness in the long term. The aims of treatment of hand burns are to protect the wound surface from infection and to provide an environment beneficial to healing (Muddiman, 1989).

1. Procedure for the care of a patient with burns to the hand on admission to the Burns Unit

It is important that burns to the hands are assessed and treated by both medical and paramedical staff who are adequately trained in burn care. Therefore, admitting the patient to the Burns Unit is recommended not only to allow for appropriate wound care but also to maximise the functional ability of the hand by intensive physiotherapy starting immediately after the burn injury occurs.

See sections 1 and 2 in Chapter 1 for advice on procedures.

Equipment

Tray/trolley
Disposable gloves
Doppler machine (optional)
PVC (cling film)
Burns assessment chart
Patient's prescription chart
Nursing documentation charts

Action	Rationale
On admission of the patient to the Burns Unit obtain a detailed history of the injury e.g. cause and duration of contact of the source.	To assist in ascertaining the severity of the injury. History allows for appropriate interventions to be performed (Kemble and Lamb, 1987).
Determine if any first aid treatment has been carried out and what type.	To assess whether appropriate interventions have been performed.
Ask the patient if he or she has any pain, noting quality and intensity. Administer analgesia as prescribed by the medical staff.	To minimise pain and discomfort for the patient.

Action	Rationale
Apply unsterile gloves.	To protect the nurse from body fluids and minimise the risk of cross infection (Wilson, 1992).
Remove any jewellery e.g. rings, bracelets, circumferentially surrounding the extremity.	With the oedema formation that follows a burn injury, circumferential pressure may reduce perfusion and cause tissue damage.
Perform a physical inspection of the hand(s). Observe:	To assess the severity of the burn injury (Martin, 1991).
– Integrity of the skin and note exposure of any underlying structures, e.g. tendons, joints, muscles.	
– Extent of skin loss and/or presence of blisters.	To determine the percentage body surface area of the burn. The hand is usually estimated at 1% (Wilson, Fowler and Housden, 1987).
– Cyanosis/pallor of the fingers/hand. – Absent or diminishing pulses.	Cyanosis/pallor, absent or weak pulse, numbness and if the hand is cool are all indications that an escharotomy may be required to accommodate the swelling and permit blood flow to the distal area (Konop, 1991).
N.B. The use of a doppler machine may be advocated if pulses are difficult to palpate.	To confirm the presence/absence of pulses.
– If the hand/fingers are warm or cool. – Presence of pain, tingling sensation or numbness.	A cool hand/fingers, tingling or numbness indicate poor circulation of blood to the area and may indicate that an escharotomy may be required to permit blood flow to the area (Konop, 1991).
– Apply gentle counterpressure to the burn areas and note capillary refill.	Slow capillary refill may indicate poor circulation to the area. Superficial burns will show signs of blanching with gentle pressure.
Increase the temperature of the environment if the circulation to the hand is poor.	If the patient is cold, peripheral vessels constrict impeding blood flow.
When inspection is completed apply a layer of PVC (cling film) over the hand until the wounds have been assessed by the medical staff.	To provide a temporary non-stick dressing (Lendrum and Bowden-Jones, 1976; Wilson and French, 1987; Milner, 1988) until the prescribed dressings are applied.
	PVC film contains no antimicrobial agents, it is therefore not advocated as a long-term dressing (Davies, 1983).

Action	Rationale
Elevate the hand in a Bradford sling (above the level of the heart) well supported by pillows under the upper arm.	To relieve venous congestion and minimise the collection of oedema (Sykes and Bailey, 1975). If unsupported, nerve damage can occur due to the sling cutting into the arm.
Record the history and physical examination in the appropriate documentation.	To maintain an accurate record.
Continue to monitor and record circulation to fingertips, noting warmth, colour, pulses and sensation. Inform medical staff immediately of any abnormalities.	To detect early signs of complications which may indicate the need for an escharotomy (Konop, 1991).
Assist the doctor with an escharotomy (see appropriate procedure) if required.	To accommodate the swelling and permit blood flow to the distal areas.

2. Procedure for applying a plastic bag to the hand

Burns to the hands can be treated very successfully by using plastic bags (Slater and Hughes, 1971) and antibacterial cream. See Figure 9.1.

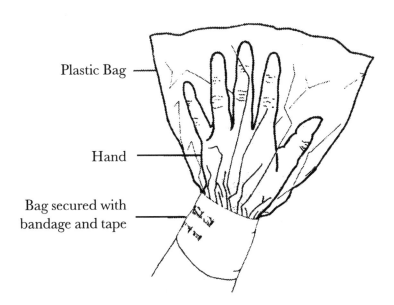

Plastic Bag

Hand

Bag secured with bandage and tape

Figure 9.1 *Hand enclosed in a plastic bag.*

Plastic bags may be indicated when the patient has a circumferential burn to the hand/fingers and circulation needs to be monitored closely.

They are easy to apply, allow for a moist environment conducive to wound healing, allow continuous visual monitoring of the hand, promote independence, and enable the patient to move the fingers freely without being restricted by bulky dressings.

According to Bailey and Desai (1973), Reid (1974), Sykes and Bailey (1975) there are disadvantages: over a period of time the antibacterial cream melts and collects in the bottom of the bag which looks unsightly and may become heavy, dragging across the burn surface and making mobilisation difficult. The skin on the hand also becomes very macerated making it difficult in some cases not only to assess which area of the hand is burned (Muddiman, 1989), but also to determine the burn size, its depth and extent of healing and hence the possible need for interventional surgery (Terrill, Kedwards and Lawrence, 1991).

In addition, plastic bags are fragile and tear easily (Martin, French and Theakstone, 1990) requiring the patient to undergo additional dressing changes and increasing the risk of infection (Muddiman, 1989).

See sections 1–5 in Chapter 1 for advice on procedures.

Equipment

Trolley
Sterile dressing pack
Sterile scissors
1 pair of sterile gloves
2 pairs of unsterile gloves
Plastic bag of appropriate size
Sachet of saline and alcohol swab
Sterile gauze swabs
Sterile towel
Crepe bandage and adhesive tape
Antibacterial cream (Silver Sulphadiazine)
Patient's prescription chart
Disposal bag
Paraffin gauze (optional)
Bacteriological wound swab (optional)
PVC (cling film)
Hand bath/bowl
Povidone Iodine aqueous solution 10% (optional)
Towel (optional)

Action	Rationale
Administer analgesia as prescribed 30 minutes prior to commencing the procedure.	To minimise pain and discomfort for the patient.
Remove hand from sling and ensure patient is in a comfortable position.	For the comfort of the patient.
Prepare the hand bath/bowl: – Fill three-quarters of the bath or bowl with warm water.	To ensure the hand bath is ready for use as soon as the old dressings are removed.

Action	Rationale
– As an option add measured amount of Povidone Iodine aqueous solution 10% to the water, and mix.	Povidone Iodine is an antibacterial solution effective in cleaning burn wounds (Brennan and Leaper, 1985). It is non irritant and has been used successfully in the treatment of burns (Garnes, 1959; Wynn-Willliams and Montalliv, 1965; Cesany, 1977; de Kock and van der Merwe, 1987).
Apply unsterile gloves.	To protect the nurse against body fluids and to minimise the risk of cross infection.
Remove the existing bag/dressing and discard in the disposal bag. If a Goretex bag send to the laundry, do not discard.	To minimise the risk of cross infection.
	Laundering removes excess cream, etc. from inside the bag, preparing it for autoclaving and further use.
Remove gloves and wash hands.	To minimise the risk of cross infection.
If the wound appears red, inflamed, smells or is oozing purulent discharge, take a bacteriological wound swab for culture and sensitivity. Label and send to the microbiology laboratory.	To detect early signs of infection that may delay healing.
Gently lower the hand into the bath/bowl and allow to soak.	The use of a hand bath will assist with wound cleansing and hand exercises.
Apply unsterile gloves and using gauze swabs gently wipe over the hand and between the fingers.	Cleansing will facilitate the removal of old creams, dead skin, etc.
Encourage the patient to perform hand exercises whilst immersing the hand in the bath.	Exercising is easier without restrictive dressings and allows free movement.
Remove the hand and dry gently with gauze or a soft towel.	
Cover the hand with PVC (cling film).	To act as a temporary dressing whilst the contents of the hand bath are disposed of. To allow time for wound assessment by medical staff (if required) (Lendrum and Bowden Jones, 1976; Davies, 1983; Wilson and French, 1987; Milner, 1988).
Remove the hand bath/bowl and contents.	To remove dirty water and to minimise the risk of spillage.
Empty the contents of the bath/bowl down the sluice/toilet.	To minimise the risk of cross infection.

Action	Rationale
Wash out the bath/bowl with hot soapy water. Rinse and dry thoroughly and return to the appropriate storage area.	To minimise the risk of cross infection.
Remove gloves and wash hands.	To minimise the risk of cross infection.
Apply sterile gloves and place the hand on the sterile towel.	To maintain asepsis.
If any further exudate is present, moisten the gauze swabs with saline and using the gloved hand gently wipe over the skin and between the fingers.	To remove any exudate, scabs or loose skin.
Using the sterile scissors, burst and deroof any blisters.	Blisters are burst as they may restrict movement and blister fluid retards healing by impairing local immunity (Rockwell and Ehrlich, 1990; Anon 1990). Deroofing the skin removes any dead tissue that may harbour micro-organisms (Lawrence, 1989) and enables the nurse to assess the depth of the wound.
Using the forceps, lift up any slough or loose dead tissue and with the sterile scissors cut as close to the skin as possible	Slough and/or dead tissue may provide a focus for micro-organisms (Lawrence 1989).
Apply a layer of antibacterial cream e.g. Silver Sulphadiazine, directly to the burn areas.	Silver Sulphadiazine cream is an antibacterial agent effective in the treatment of hand burns (Sykes and Bailey, 1975; Hoffman, 1984) which has been remarkably successful with burnt hands in particular (de Boer and Collinson, 1981).
If there are any areas of burn around the wrist apply a thin layer of Silver Sulphadiazine cream, cover with 2–3 layers of paraffin gauze and cover with gauze swabs.	To provide a separate dressing to the wrist on which to secure the plastic bag.
Even if there are no burns, apply several layers of gauze swabs around the wrist/forearm.	Gauze will absorb some of the exudate that may run down into the wrist area when the hands are elevated (Slater and Hughes, 1971; Terrill, Kedwards and Lawrence, 1991).
Ask the patient to place the hand inside the plastic bag.	To encourage co-operation of the patient and to apply the bag over the hand.

Action	Rationale
Remove any excess air and ensure the patient has enough room to spread the fingers.	Excess air causes the bag to bulge under tension and restricts the patient from using the hand to pick up objects, e.g. cup, knife, fork.
Gather the bag at the wrist/forearm and secure over the gauze with crepe bandage and adhesive tape.	To absorb any excess exudate and to secure the bag in place (Slater and Hughes, 1971).
Apply splint(s) over the bag if required, on advice of medical staff and/or physiotherapist.	To allow for correct positioning of the hand.
Elevate hand(s) in slings with upper arm(s) well supported by pillows.	To relieve venous congestion and minimise the collection of oedema (Sykes and Bailey, 1975).
Record in the appropriate documentation.	To maintain an accurate record.
Repeat the procedure on a daily basis or more often if the bag bursts or becomes full of exudate.	To allow for continual wound assessment and evaluation of treatment. For the comfort of the patient.
Encourage active and passive exercises of the hand and fingers throughout the day, involving a physiotherapist as required.	Exercise maintains joint mobility, reduces stiffness and oedema (Muddiman, 1989) and strengthens muscle tone. The physiotherapist may be involved in giving advice to patients on an exercise regime.
Encourage the patient to use the hand for feeding and drinking as much as possible involving the physiotherapist as required.	To maintain independence and increase self-esteem.
If the burns are circumferential, monitor and record the circulation of the fingers noting warmth, colour, pulses and sensation 1–4 hourly as directed by medical staff and inform them immediately if there are any abnormalities.	To indicate signs of complications. A plastic bag allows for these observations to be made while the bag is still *in situ* (Sykes and Bailey, 1975). Impaired circulation may indicate the need for an escharotomy to be performed (Konop, 1991).

3. Procedure for applying a Goretex bag to the hand

Burns to the hand can be treated very successfully with Goretex bags or mittens and antibacterial cream (Terrill, Kedwards and Lawrence, 1991).

Goretex is a thin membrane made from expanded polytetrafluoroethylene (PTFE) teflon. It is vapour permeable and acts as a barrier to airborne particles and bacteria (Muddiman, 1989). Goretex is opaque and is preferred by patients and their relatives as it is less distressing for them not to see the burned hand (Terrill, Kedwards and

Lawrence, 1991). Goretex bags are comparable to plastic bags in respect of healing, comfort, mobilisation, ease of use and the degree of swelling that occurs but prove to be superior in reducing skin maceration (Terrill, Kedwards and Lawrence, 1991), allowing easier assessment of burn areas, requiring fewer bag changes, being more robust and not causing exudate to pool in the bottom (Martin, French and Theakstone, 1990).

From the physiotherapist's point of view Goretex bags allow free, comfortable exercise, unencumbered by the weight of accumulated exudate. Patients are more confident using the hand as they are able to grip objects securely as the bag is non slip and splints may be applied easily over the bags (Terrill, Kedwards and Lawrence, 1991).

However, they do have limitations; they are not transparent and are therefore not advised for use in circumferential burns. High costs are initially involved in purchasing the material but this is offset by the reduced number of dressings and commitment of nursing time (Muddiman, 1989; Martin, French and Theakstone, 1990).

When the bags are removed, they are sent to the laundry to be washed then autoclaved by the central sterile services department (CSSD) and returned to the unit individually packed.

Goretex has been made into both bags and mittens of varying sizes. Appropriate type and size should be selected on an individual basis.

See sections 1–5 in Chapter 1 for advice on procedures.

Equipment

Trolley
Sterile dressing pack
Sterile scissors
1 pair of sterile gloves
2 pairs of unsterile gloves
Goretex bag or mitten (of appropriate size)
Sachet of saline and alcohol swab
Sterile gauze swabs
Sterile towel
Crepe bandage and adhesive tape
Antibacterial cream, (Silver Sulphadiazine)
Patient's prescription chart
Disposal bag
Paraffin gauze (optional)
Bacteriological wound swab (optional)
PVC (cling film)
Hand bath/bowl
Povidone Iodine aqueous solution 10% (optional)
Towel (optional)

Action	Rationale
Administer analgesia as prescribed 30 minutes prior to commencing the procedure.	To minimise pain and discomfort for the patient.
Remove hand from sling and ensure the patient is in a comfortable position.	For the comfort of the patient.
Prepare the hand bath/bowl.	To ensure the hand bath/bowl is ready for use as soon as the old dressings are removed.
– Fill three-quarters of the bath or bowl with warm water.	
– Optionally add measured amount of Povidone Iodine aqueous solution 10% to the water and mix.	Povidone Iodine is an antibacterial solution effective in cleaning burn wounds (Brennan and Leaper, 1985; Martin, French and Theakstone, 1990). It is non irritant and has been used successfully in the treatment of burns (Garnes, 1959; Wynn Williams and Montalliv, 1965; Cesany, 1977; de Kocke and van der Merwe, 1987).
Apply unsterile gloves.	For the protection of the nurse against body fluids and to minimise the risk of cross infection.
Remove the existing bag/dressing and discard in disposal bag. If a Goretex bag send to the laundry, do not discard.	Laundering removes excess cream from inside the bag, preparing it for autoclaving and further use.
Remove gloves and wash hands.	To minimise the risk of cross infection.
If the wound appears red, inflamed, smells, or is oozing purulent discharge take a bacteriological wound swab for culture and sensitivity. Label and send to the microbiology laboratory.	To detect early signs of infection that may delay healing.
Gently lower the hand into the bath/bowl and allow to soak.	Use of a hand bath/bowl will assist with wound cleansing and hand exercises.
Apply unsterile gloves and using gauze swabs gently wipe over the hand and in between the fingers.	Cleansing will facilitate the removal of old cream, dead skin, etc.
Encourage the patient to perform hand exercises whilst immersing the hand in the bath.	Exercising is easier without restrictive dressings and allows free movement.
Remove the hand and dry gently with gauze or a soft towel.	

Action	Rationale
Cover the hand with PVC (cling film).	To act as a temporary dressing while the contents of the bath/bowl are disposed of. To allow time for wound assessment by medical staff (if required) (Lendrum and Bowden Jones, 1976, Davies, 1983; Wilson and French, 1987, Milner, 1988).
Remove the hand bath/bowl(s) (and contents).	To remove dirty water and to minimise the risk of spillage.
Empty the contents of the bath/bowl(s) down the sluice/toilet.	To minimise the risk of cross infection.
Wash out the bath/bowl(s) with hot soapy water. Rinse and dry thoroughly and return to the appropriate storage area.	To minimise the risk of cross infection.
Remove gloves and wash hands.	To minimise the risk of cross infection.
Apply sterile gloves and place hand(s) on the sterile towel.	To maintain asepsis.
If any further exudate is present, moisten the gauze swabs with saline and using the gloved hand, gently wipe over the skin on the hand and between the fingers.	To remove any exudate, scabs or loose skin.
Using the sterile scissors, burst and deroof any blisters.	Blisters are burst as they may restrict movement and blister fluid retards healing by impairment of local immunity (Rockwell and Ehrlich, 1990; Anon, 1990). Deroofing the skin removes any dead tissue that may harbour micro-organisms (Lawrence, 1989) and enables the nurse to assess the depth of the wound.
Using the forceps, lift up any slough or loose or dead tissue and with the sterile scissors cut as close to the skin as possible.	Slough and/or dead tissue may provide a focus for micro-organisms (Lawrence, 1989)
Apply a layer of antibacterial cream, e.g. Silver Sulphadiazine cream directly to the burn areas.	Silver Sulphadiazine cream is an anti-bacterial agent effective in the treatment of burns, (Terrill, Kedwards, Lawrence, 1991; Fox, 1968; Stanford et al., 1969; Hoffman, 1984) which has been remarkably successful with burnt hands in particular (de Boer and Collinson, 1981).

Action	Rationale
If there are any areas of burn around the wrist apply a thin layer of Silver Sulphadiazine cream, cover with 2–3 layers of paraffin gauze and cover with gauze swabs.	To provide a separate dressing to the wrist on which to secure the Goretex bag/mitten.
Even if there are no burns, apply several layers of gauze swabs around the wrist/forearm.	Gauze will absorb some of the exudate that may run down into the wrist area when the hands are elevated (Slater and Hughes, 1971; Terrill, Kedwards and Lawrence, 1991).
Ask the patient to place the hand inside the Goretex bag/mitten.	To encourage co-operation of the patient and to apply the bag over the hand (Martin, French and Theakstone, 1990). Goretex bags offer a means of reducing the amount of accumulated exudate and hand maceration (Terrill, Kedwards and Lawrence, 1991).
Ensure the patient has enough room to spread the fingers.	To avoid poor positioning of the hand inside the bag/mitten and not to restrict the patient from using the hand.
Gather the bag at the wrist/forearm and secure over the gauze by pulling the cord and tying in a bow or with crepe bandage and adhesive tape.	To secure the bag in place — cords allow for the bag to be secured on the wrist and minimise the use of extra bandages. Tape is preferable to pins for the safety of the patient.
Apply splint(s) over the bag if required on advice of medical staff and/or physiotherapist.	To allow for correct positioning of the hand (Martin, French and Theakstone, 1990; Terrill, Kedwards and Lawrence, 1991).
Elevate hand(s) in slings with upper arms well supported by pillows	To relieve venous congestion and minimise the collection of oedema (Sykes and Bailey, 1975).
Record in the appropriate documentation.	To maintain an accurate record.
Repeat the procedure on a daily basis or more often if required.	To allow for continual wound assessment and evaluation of treatment. For the comfort of the patient.
Throughout the day encourage active and passive exercises of the hand and fingers, involving the physiotherapist, as required.	Exercise maintains joint mobility and strengthens muscle tone (Martin, French and Theakstone, 1990), advice can be given to patients on an exercise regime.
N.B. For physiotherapy, the bags may need to be removed, due to their opaque nature.	To allow for adequate supervision of movement.

Action	Rationale
Encourage the patient to use the hands for feeding and drinking as much as possible.	To maintain independence and increase self-esteem. Goretex has a non-slip nature and is durable allowing confidence in gripping objects securely (Terrill, Kedwards and Lawrence, 1991).

4. Procedure for applying a dressing to the hand

Dressings to the hands are not usually applied in the initial stages of a burn injury (bags are preferable) as they reduce mobility (Muddiman, 1989). Dressings are used post surgery and as healing progresses. They should be changed every 1–2 days, which is important in minimising the development of joint stiffness and contributes to a reduction in oedema. The aims of treatment are to minimise infection, provide a moist environment for wound healing and reduce swelling, whilst not being too bulky to limit hand, and/or finger movements which may cause stiffness.

During treatment it is important to maintain a team approach with the physiotherapist and occupational therapist. Functional ability of the hand should be maximised by exercising frequently and applying splints where appropriate to avoid joint stiffness and the development of contractures in the long term.

See sections 1–5 in Chapter 1 for advice on procedures.

Equipment

Trolley
Sterile dressing pack
Sterile scissors
1 pair of sterile gloves
2 pairs of unsterile gloves
Sachet of saline and alcohol swab
Paraffin gauze
Sterile towel
Sterile gauze swabs (large)
Sterile gauze swabs (small)
Tubular bandage/elasticated tubular finger dressings (with applicator) or crepe bandage and adhesive tape
Patient's prescription chart
Antibacterial cream (Silver Sulphadiazine) (optional)
Disposal bag
PVC (cling film)
Povidone Iodine aqueous solution 10% (optional)
Towel (optional)
Bacteriological wound swab (optional)

Action	Rationale
Administer analgesia as prescribed 30 minutes prior to commencing the procedure.	To minimise pain and discomfort for the patient.
Remove hand from sling and ensure the patient is in comfortable position.	For the comfort of the patient.
Prepare the hand bath/bowl.	To ensure the hand bath/bowl is ready for use as soon as the dressings are removed.
– Fill three-quarters of the bath or bowl with warm water.	
– As an option add measured amount of Povidone Iodine aqueous solution 10% to the water and mix.	Povidone Iodine is an antibacterial solution effective in cleaning burn wounds (Brennan and Leaper, 1985) It is non irritant and has been used successfully for the treatment of burns (Garnes, 1959; Wynn-Williams and Montalliv, 1965; Cesany, 1977; de Kocke and van der Merwe, 1987).
Apply unsterile gloves.	For the protection of the nurse against body fluids and to minimise the risk of cross infection.
Remove existing dressing (leaving any gauze that is adherent) and discard in the disposal bag.	To minimise the risk of additional trauma caused by removing dressings that are adherent.
Remove gloves and wash hands.	To minimise the risk of cross infection.
If the wound appears red, inflamed, smells, or is oozing purulent discharge take a bacteriological wound swab for culture and sensitivity. Label and send to the microbiology laboratory.	To detect early signs of infection that may delay healing.
Gently lower the hand into the bath/bowl and allow to soak.	Use of a hand bath will allow adherent dressings to be soaked off to minimise pain and assist with wound cleansing.
Apply unsterile gloves and using gauze swabs gently wipe over the hand and in between the fingers.	Cleansing will facilitate the removal of old cream, dead skin, etc.
Encourage the patient to perform hand exercises whilst immersing the hand in the bath/bowl.	Exercising is easier without restrictive dressings and allows free movement.
Remove hand and dry gently with gauze or a soft towel.	

Action	Rationale
Cover the hand with PVC (cling film).	To act as a temporary dressing while the contents of the hand bath are disposed of and to allow time for wound assessment by medical staff (if required) (Lendrum and Bowden Jones, 1976; Davies, 1983; Wilson and French, 1987; Milner, 1988).
Remove the hand bath/bowl(s) (and contents).	To remove dirty water and to minimise the risk of spillage.
Empty the contents of the bath/bowl(s) down the sluice/toilet.	To minimise the risk of cross infection.
Wash out the bath/bowl(s) with hot soapy water. Rinse and dry thoroughly and return to the appropriate storage area.	To minimise the risk of cross infection.
Remove gloves and wash hands.	To minimise the risk of cross infection.
Apply sterile gloves and place the hand on the sterile towel.	To maintain asepsis.
If any exudate is present, moisten the gauze swabs with saline and, using the gloved hand, gently wipe over the skin and in between the fingers.	To remove any exudate, scabs or loose skin.
Using sterile scissors, burst and deroof any blisters.	Blisters are burst as they may restrict movement and blister fluid retards healing by impairing local immunity (Rockwell and Ehrlich, 1990; Anon, 1990). Deroofing the skin removes any dead skin that may harbour micro-organisms (Lawrence, 1989) and enables the nurse to assess the depth of the wound.
Using forceps lift up any slough or loose dead tissue and using the sterile scissors cut as close to the skin as possible.	Slough and/or dead tissue may provide a focus for micro-organisms (Lawrence, 1989).
N.B. With burns to the fingers, treat and apply dressings to each digit separately.	Prevents adherence of one wound surface to another which may cause webbing. May also facilitate easier movement.
Apply a layer of anti-bacterial cream, e.g. Silver Sulphadiazine cream directly to the burn areas.	Silver Sulphadiazine cream is an antimicrobial agent effective in the treatment of burn (Sykes and Bailey, 1975; Hoffman, 1984) which has been remarkably successful with burnt hands in particular (de Boer and Collinson, 1981).

Action	Rationale
Cover with 2–3 layers of paraffin gauze and cover with gauze swabs (small sizes are available for use on fingers).	Paraffin gauze is a bleached cotton gauze impregnated with Vaseline — it provides a nonstick dressing and a moist environment for wound healing (Thomas, 1994), gauze swabs are used to absorb exudate.
Avoid wrapping the paraffin gauze and gauze swabs circumferentially around the finger(s).	As oedema forms or drainage saturates the gauze and dries, constriction may result and the circulation becomes impaired.
With dressings to the hand apply crepe bandage and secure with adhesive tape.	To secure dressings in place. Tape is preferable to pins for the safety of the patient.
With dressings to the fingers: using the appropriate size applicator and/or elasticated tubular bandage, apply separate finger dressings.	To secure dressings in place, and allow for individual finger exercises to be performed.
Apply splint(s) over the dressings if required.	To allow for correct positioning of the hand.
Elevate hand in a sling with upper arm supported by pillows.	To relieve venous congestion and minimise the collection of oedema (Sykes and Bailey, 1975).
Record in the appropriate documentation.	To maintain an accurate record.
Repeat the procedure on a daily basis or more often as directed by medical staff	To allow for continual wound assessment and evaluation of treatment. Twice daily dressings may be required if wounds are infected, leaking or require intense physiotherapy.
Throughout the day encourage active and passive exercises of the hand and fingers.	Exercise maintains joint mobility and strengthens muscle tone.
Encourage the patient to use the hands for feeding, drinking and assisting with other daily living activities as much as possible.	To maintain independence.

References

Anon (1990) Should burn blisters be burst? Emergency Medicine 22 (1): 57–9.

Bailey BN, Desai SN (1973) An approach to the treatment of hand burns. Injury 4: 335.

Brennan SS, Leaper DJ (1985) The effects of antiseptics on the healing wound. British Journal of Surgery 72: 780–82.

Cesany P (1977) Clinical experience with povidone iodine (Betadine) in the treatment of burns and as an adjunct in plastic surgery. Pharmatherapeutica 1: 514.

Davies JLW (1983) Synthetic materials for covering burn wounds. Progress towards perfection. Part 1. Short term dressing material. Burns Journal. 10: 94.

de Boer P, Collinson PO (1981) The use of silver sulphadiazine occlusive dressings for finger-tip injuries. The Journal of Bone and Joint Surgery. 63-B (4): 545–7.

de Kocke M, van der Merwe AE (1987) A study to assess the effects of a new Betadine cream formulation compared to a standard topical treatment regimen for burns. Burns Journal 13 (1): 69–74.

Fox CL (1968) Silver sulphadiazine — A new topical therapy for pseudomonas in burns. Archives of Surgery, 96: 18.

Garnes AL (1959) Clinical evaluation of povidone iodine in surgical practice. American Journal of Surgery. 97: 49.

Hoffman S (1984) Silver sulphadiazine cream: an antibacterial agent for topical use in burns. A review of the literature. Scandinavian Journal of Plastic and Reconstructive Surgery 18: 18, 119.

Kemble JVH, Lamb B (1984) Plastic Surgical and Burns Nursing. Gloucester: Baillière Tindall.

Kemble JV, Lamb BE (1987) Practical Burns Management. London: Hodder and Stoughton.

Konop DJ (1991) General local treatment. In Trofino RB (Ed) Nursing Care of the Burn Injured Patient, Philadelphia: FA Davis Company. pp 55–6.

Lawrence JC (1989) Management of burns. The Dressing Times 2 (3): 1–4.

Lendrum J, Bowden-Jones E (1976) A new dressing for burns. Enclosure in a plasticised polyvinyl sheet. Burns Journal 2: 86.

Martin MT (1991) Burns of the hands and feet. In Trofino RB (Ed) Nursing Care of the Burn Injured Patient Philadelphia: FA Davis Company. pp 212–21.

Martin DL, French GWG, Theakstone J (1990) The use of semi-permeable membranes for wound management. British Journal of Plastic Surgery. 43: 55–60.

Milner RH (1988) Plasticised polyvinylchloride film as a temporary burns dressing — a microbiological study. Burns Journal 14 (1): 62–5.

Muddiman R (1989) A new concept in hand burn dressing. Nursing Standard (Special Supplement) September 23: 1–3.

Reid WH (1974) Care of the burned hand. Hand 6: 163.

Rockwell C, Ehrlich D (1990) Should burn blisters be burst? Journal of Burn Care and Rehabilitation 11: 93.

Slater RM, Hughes NC (1971) A simplified method of treating burns of the hands. British Journal of Plastic Surgery 24: 296.

Stanford W, Rappole BW, Fox CL et al., (1969) Clinical experience with silver sulphadiazine. Journal of Trauma, 9: 377.

Sykes PJ, Bailey BN (1975) Treatment of hand burns with occlusive dressings. A comparison of three methods. Burns Journal, 2: 162–8.

Terrill PJ, Kedwards SM, Lawrence JC (1991) The use of Goretex bags for hand burns. Burns Journal. 17 (2): 161–5.

Thomas S (1994) Jelonet. In Thomas S (Ed) Handbook of Wound Dressings. London: MacMillan. pp 98–9.

Wilson J (1992) Theory and practice of isolation nursing. Nursing Standard (17): 30–1.

Wilson GR, Fowler CA, Housden PL (1987) A new burn area assessment chart. Burns Journal 13 (5): 401–5.

Wilson G, French G (1987) Plasticised polyvinylchloride as a temporary dressing for burns. British Medical Journal 294: 556–7.

Wynn Williams D, Montalliv G (1965) The effects of povidone iodine in the treatment of burns and traumatic losses of skin. Journal of Plastic Surgery 18: 146.

Chapter 10
Care of patient with burns to the feet

Burns to the feet may occur as a result of electricity, frostbite, chemicals, flames or scalds.

Except for the soles, feet have a thin epidermal and dermal layer of skin protecting a complex structure of nerves, tendons, muscles and bones. Therefore, any tissue damage may easily expose these structures (Martin, 1991). Because of the unique and important anatomical structure of the feet, their functional importance and their sensory role, burn injuries to the feet affect mobility and have long-term implications for rehabilitation (Martin, 1991). General care of burns to the feet is to provide continual wound assessment, to minimise infection, to remove dead tissue, to provide an environment conducive to wound healing, to reduce swelling and to preserve function.

When burns to the feet/toes are circumferential it is recommended that a plastic bag is applied initially to allow for close monitoring of the circulation. Once this is established, the application of Goretex bags or alternative dressings is recommended. Function is maintained through active and passive exercises and appropriate positioning of the feet, and lymphatic and venous drainage is promoted by elevating the feet.

With fill thickness burns early excision and skin grafting within 3–4 days post injury is advised to enable early mobilisation and rehabilitation.

1. Procedure for the case of a patient with burns to the foot on admission to the Burns Unit

It is important that burns to the feet are assessed and treated by both medical and nursing staff who are adequately trained in burns care. Obtaining an accurate history of the accident will assist in determining the cause of the burn as well as length of contact of the source with the skin, which will be reflected in the depth of the burn injury. The feet have great functional importance for patients affecting mobility. Admitting the patient to the Burns Unit allows for appropriate wound care and intensive physiotherapy to minimise long-term complications.

See sections 1 and 2 in Chapter 1 for advice on procedures.

Equipment

Tray/trolley.
Disposable gloves
Doppler machine (optional)
PVC (cling film)
Burns assessment chart
Patient's prescription chart
Nursing documentation charts

Action	Rationale
On admission of the patient to the Burns Unit obtain a detailed history of the injury, e.g. cause and duration of contact with the source.	To assist in ascertaining the severity of the injury. History allows for appropriate interventions to be performed (Kemble and Lamb, 1987).
Determine if any first aid treatment has been carried out and what type.	To assess whether appropriate interventions have been performed.
Ask the patient if he or she has any pain, noting quality and intensity. Administer analgesia as described by the medical staff.	To minimise pain and discomfort for patient.
Apply unsterile gloves.	To protect the nurse from body fluids and minimise the risk of cross infection (Wilson, 1992).
Perform a physical inspection of the feet. Observe:	To assess the severity of the burn injury (Martin, 1991).
– Integrity of the skin and note exposure of any underlying structures, e.g. tendons, joints, muscles.	
– Extent of skin loss and/or presence of blisters.	To determine the percentage body surface area of the burn (Wilson, Fowler and Housden, 1987).
– Cyanosis/pallor of the toes/foot. – Absent or diminishing pulses. **N.B. The use of a Doppler machine may be advocated if pulses are difficult to palpate.** – If the foot/toes are warm or cool. – Presence of pain, tingling sensation, numbness.	Cyanosis/pallor, absent or weak pulse, numbness and coolness of the foot are all indications that an escharotomy may be required to accommodate the swelling and permit blood flow to the distal area (Konop, 1991). A Doppler machine will confirm the presence or absence of pulses.
– Apply gentle counterpressure to the burn areas and note capillary refill.	Slow capillary refill may indicate poor circulation to the area. Superficial burns will show signs of blanching with gentle pressure.

Action	Rationale
Increase the temperature of the environment if the circulation to the foot is poor.	If the patient is cold peripheral vessels constrict impeding blood flow.
When inspection is complete, apply a layer of PVC (cling film) over the foot until the wounds have been assessed by the medical staff.	To provide a temporary non-stick dressing (Lendrum and Bowden Jones, 1976; Wilson and French, 1987; Milner, 1988) until the prescribed dressings are applied. The PVC film contains no antimicrobial agents and is therefore not advocated for long-term use (Davies, 1983).
Elevate the foot and ensure it is well supported by pillows.	To relieve venous congestion and minimise the collection of oedema.
Record the history and physical examination in the appropriate documentation.	To maintain an accurate record.
Continue to monitor and record circulation to the toes, noting warmth, colour, pulses and sensation. Inform the doctor immediately of any abnormalities.	To detect early signs of complications. May indicate the need for an escharotomy (Konop, 1991).
Assist the doctor with an escharotomy (see appropriate procedure) if required.	To accommodate the swelling and permit blood flow to the distal areas.

2. Procedure for applying a plastic bag to the foot

Burns to the foot can be treated very successfully with plastic bags (Slater and Hughes, 1971) and antibacterial cream. Plastic bags may be indicated for use when the patient has a circumferential burn to the foot/toes and circulation needs to be monitored closely. They are easy to apply, create a moist environment conducive to wound healing, allow continuous visual monitoring of the foot, promote independence and enable the patient to move the toes freely without being restricted by bulky dressings.

According to Bailey and Desai (1973), Reid (1974) and Sykes and Bailey (1975) there are disadvantages: over a period of time the antibacterial cream melts and collects in the bottom of the bag which looks unsightly and may become heavy making mobilisation difficult. The skin on the foot/toes becomes very macerated making it difficult in some cases to assess not only which area of the foot is burned (Muddiman, 1989), but also the burn size, its depth, the extent of healing and the possible need for interventional surgery (Terrill, Kedwards and Lawrence, 1991).

It is *not* advisable to allow the patient to walk in the bags as they are fragile and tear easily (Martin, French and Theakstone, 1990). The patient is also at risk of slipping on the cream inside the bag during mobilisation. Frequent dressing changes increase the risk of infection (Muddiman, 1989).

See sections 1–5 in Chapter 1 for advice on procedures.

Equipment

Trolley
Sterile dressing pack
Sterile scissors
1 pair of sterile gloves
2 pairs of unsterile gloves
Plastic bag of appropriate size
Sachet of saline and alcohol swab
Sterile gauze swabs
Sterile towel
Crepe bandage and adhesive tape
Antibacterial cream (Silver Sulphadiazine).
Patient's prescription chart
Disposal bag
Paraffin gauze (optional)
Bacteriological wound swab (optional)
PVC (cling film)
Foot bath/bowl
Povidone Iodine aqueous solution 10% (optional)
Towel (optional)

Action	Rationale
Administer analgesia as prescribed 30 minutes prior to commencing the procedure.	To minimise pain and discomfort for the patient.
Remove pillows from under the patient's feet and ensure the patient is in a comfortable position.	For the comfort of the patient.
Prepare the foot bath/bowl - Fill three-quarters of the bath or bowl with warm water.	To ensure the foot bath is ready for use as soon as the old dressings are removed.
- As an option add measured amount of Povidone Iodine aqueous solution 10% to the water and mix.	Povidone Iodine is an antibacterial solution effective in cleaning burn wounds (Brennan and Leaper, 1985). It is non irritant and has been used successfully in the treatment of burns (Garnes, 1959; Wynn Williams and Montalliv, 1965; Cesany, 1977; de Kocke and van der Merwe, 1987).
Apply unsterile gloves.	For the protection of the nurse against body fluids and to minimise the risk of cross infection.

Action	Rationale
Remove the existing bag/dressing and discard in the disposal bag. If a Goretex bag send to the laundry, do not discard.	To minimise the risk of cross infection. Laundering the Goretex bag will remove excess cream and prepare it for autoclaving and further use.
Remove gloves and wash hands.	To minimise the risk of cross infection.
If the wound appears red, inflamed, smells, or is oozing purulent discharge take a bacteriological wound swab for culture and sensitivity. Label and send to the microbiology laboratory.	To detect early signs of infection that may delay healing.
Gently lower the foot into the bath/bowl and allow to soak.	The use of a foot bath will assist with wound cleansing and foot exercises.
Apply unsterile gloves and using gauze swabs gently wipe over the foot and in between the toes.	Cleansing will facilitate the removal of old cream, dead skin, etc.
Encourage the patient to perform ankle exercises whilst immersing the foot in the bath.	Exercising is easier without restrictive dressings and allows free movement.
Remove the foot and dry gently with gauze or a soft towel.	
Cover the foot with PVC (cling film).	To act as a temporary dressing while the contents of the foot bath are disposed of. To allow time for wound assessment by medical staff (if required) (Lendrum and Bowden Jones, 1976; Davies, 1983; Wilson and French, 1987; Milner, 1988).
Remove the bath/bowl(s) and contents away from the patient.	To remove dirty water and minimise the risk of spillage.
Empty the contents of the bath/bowl(s) down the sluice/toilet.	To minimise the risk of cross infection.
Wash out the bath/bowl(s) with hot soapy water. Rinse and dry thoroughly and return to the appropriate storage area.	To minimise the risk of cross infection.
Remove gloves and wash hands.	To minimise the risk of cross infection.
Apply sterile gloves and place foot on the sterile towel.	To maintain asepsis.
If any further exudate is present, moisten the gauze swabs with saline and using the gloved hand, gently wipe over the skin and in between the toes.	To remove any exudate, scabs or loose skin.

Action	Rationale
Apply a layer of antibacterial cream, e.g. Silver Sulphadiazine cream directly to the burn areas.	Silver Sulphadiazine cream is an antimicrobial agent effective in treatment of burns (Hoffman, 1984).
If there are any areas of burn around the ankle apply a thin layer of Silver Sulphadiazine cream, cover with 2–3 layers of paraffin gauze and cover with gauze swabs.	To provide a separate dressing to the ankle on which to secure the plastic bag.
Even if there are no burns in that area still apply several layers of gauze swabs around the ankle.	Gauze will absorb some of the exudate that may run down into the ankle area when the foot is elevated (Terrill, Kedwards and Lawrence, 1991).
Ask the patient to place the foot inside the plastic bag.	To encourage co-operation of the patient and to apply the bag over the foot.
Remove any excess air and ensure the patient has enough room to spread the toes.	Excess air causes the bag to bulge under tension making it more liable to burst.
Gather the bag at the ankle and secure over the gauze with crepe bandage and adhesive tape	To secure the bag in place. Tape is preferable to pins for the safety of the patient.
Apply splint(s) over the bag if required on advice of medical staff and a physiotherapist.	To allow for correct positioning of the foot to minimise the risk of foot-drop.
Elevate the foot on pillows, avoid leg dangling and weight bearing.	To relieve venous congestion and to minimise the collection of oedema (Sykes and Bailey, 1975).
Record in the appropriate documentation.	To maintain an accurate record.
Repeat the procedure on a daily basis or more often if the bag bursts or becomes full of exudate.	To allow for continual wound assessment and evaluation of treatment.
Throughout the day, encourage active and passive exercises of the ankle and toes involving the physiotherapist.	Exercise maintains joint mobility and strengthens muscle tone. Advice can be given to patients on an exercise regime.
If the burns are circumferential, monitor and record the circulation of the toes noting warmth, colour, pulses and sensation 1–4 hourly as directed by the medical staff and inform them immediately if there are any abnormalities.	To indicate signs of complications. A plastic bag allows for these observations to be made while the bag is *in situ* (Sykes and Bailey, 1975). Impaired circulation may indicate the need for an escharotomy to be performed (Konop, 1991).

3. Procedure for applying a Goretex bag to the foot

Burns to the foot can be treated very successfully with Goretex bags and antibacterial cream (Terrill, Kedwards and Lawrence, 1991)

Goretex is a thin membrane made from expanded polytetrafluoroethylene (PTFE) teflon. It is vapour permeable and acts as a barrier to airborne particles and bacteria (Muddiman, 1989). Goretex is opaque and is preferred by patients and their relatives as it is less distressing for them to see the burn wound to the foot. Goretex bags are comparable to plastic bags in respect of healing, comfort, mobilisation, ease of use and degree of swelling but prove to be superior in reducing maceration (Terrill Kedwards and Lawrence, 1991), allowing easier assessment of burn areas, requiring less bag changes, being more robust and not causing exudate to pool in the bottom. (Martin, French and Theakstone, 1990).

However, they do have limitations; they are not transparent and are therefore not advised for use in circumferential burns. High costs are initially involved purchasing the material but this is offset by the reduced number of dressings and commitment of nursing time (Muddiman, 1989; Martin, French and Theakstone, 1990).

When the bags are removed, they are sent to the laundry to be washed then autoclaved by the Central Sterile Services Department (CSSD) and returned to the unit individually packed.

Goretex bags are available in a choice of sizes and should be selected on an individual basis.

See section 1–5 in Chapter 1 for advice on procedures.

Equipment

Trolley
Sterile dressing pack
Sterile scissors
1 pair of sterile gloves
2 pairs of unsterile gloves
Goretex bag (of appropriate size)
Sachet of saline and alcohol swab
Sterile gauze swabs
Sterile towel
Crepe bandage and adhesive tape
Antibacterial cream (Silver Sulphadiazine)
Patient's prescription chart
Disposal bag
Paraffin gauze (optional)
PVC (cling film)
Bacteriological wound swab (optional)
Foot bath/bowl
Povidone Iodine aqueous solution 10% (optional)
Towel (optional)

Action	Rationale
Administer analgesia as prescribed 30 minutes prior to commencing the procedure.	To minimise pain and discomfort for the patient.
Remove the pillows from under the feet and ensure the patient is in a comfortable position.	For the comfort of the patient.
Prepare the foot bath/bowl.	To ensure the foot bath/bowl is ready for use as soon as the old dressings are removed.
– Fill three-quarters of the bath or bowl with warm water.	
– As an option add measured amount of Povidone Iodine aqueous solution 10% to the water and mix.	Povidone Iodine is an antibacterial solution effective in cleaning burn wounds (Brennan and Leaper, 1985; Martin, French and Theakstone, 1990), it is non irritant and has been used successfully in the treatment of burns (Garnes, 1959; Wynn Williams and Montalliv, 1965).
Apply unsterile gloves.	For the protection of the nurse against body fluids and to minimise the risk of cross infection.
Remove the existing bag/dressing and discard in disposal bag. If a Goretex bag, send to laundry, do not discard.	To minimise the risk of cross infection.
	Laundering the Goretex bag will remove excess cream and prepare it for autoclaving and further use.
Remove gloves and wash hands.	To minimise the risk of cross infection.
If the wound appears red, inflamed, smells, or is oozing purulent discharge take a bacteriological wound swab for culture and sensitivity. Label and send to the microbiology laboratory.	To detect early signs of infection that may delay healing.
Gently lower the foot into the bath/bowl and allow to soak.	Use of a foot bath will assist with wound cleansing and foot exercises.
Apply unsterile gloves and using gauze swabs gently wipe over the foot and in between the toes.	Cleansing will facilitate the removal of old cream, dead skin, etc.
Encourage the patient to perform ankle exercises whilst immersing the foot in the bath.	Exercising is easier without restrictive dressings and allows free movement.
Remove the foot and dry gently with gauze or a soft towel.	

Action	Rationale
Cover the foot with PVC (cling film).	To act as a temporary dressing while the contents of the foot bath are disposed of. To allow time for wound assessment by medical staff (if required) (Lendrum and Bowden Jones, 1976; Davies, 1983; Wilson and French, 1987; Milner, 1988).
Remove the bath/bowl(s) and contents away from the patient.	To remove dirty water and to minimise the risk of spillage
Empty the contents of the bath/bowl(s) down the sluice.	To minimise the risk of cross infection.
Wash out the bath/bowl(s) with hot soapy water. Rinse and dry thoroughly and return to the appropriate storage area.	To minimise the risk of cross infection.
Remove gloves and wash hands.	To minimise the risk of cross infection.
Apply sterile gloves and place foot on the sterile towel.	To maintain asepsis.
If any further exudate is present, moisten the gauze swabs with saline and using the gloved hand, gently wipe over the skin and in between the toes.	To remove any exudate, scabs or loose skin.
Using the sterile scissors, burst and deroof any blisters.	Blisters are burst as they may restrict movement and may cause discomfort for the patient. Blister fluid retards healing by impairment of local immunity (Rockwell and Ehrlich, 1990; Anon, 1990). Deroofing the skin removes any dead tissues that may harbour micro-organisms (Lawrence, 1989) and enables the nurse to assess the depth of the wound.
Using forceps, lift up any slough or loose dead tissue and with the sterile scissors cut as close to the skin as possible.	Slough and/or dead tissue may provide a focus for micro-organisms. (Lawrence, 1989)
Apply a layer of antibacterial cream, e.g. Silver Sulphadiazine cream directly to the burn areas.	Silver Sulphadiazine cream is an antimicrobial agent effective in the treatment of burns (Hoffman, 1984; Fox, 1968; Stanford, Rapole and Fox, 1969; Lowbury et al., 1971; Richards and Mahlangu, 1981; Pegg, 1982; Van Seane et al., 1987).

Action	Rationale
If there are any areas of burn around the ankle apply a thin layer of Silver Sulphadiazine cream, cover with 2–3 layers of paraffin gauze and cover with gauze swabs.	To provide a separate dressing to the ankle on which to secure the Goretex bag.
Even if there are no burns in that area still apply several layers of gauze swabs around the ankle.	Gauze will absorb some of the exudate that may run down into the ankle area when the foot is elevated (Terrill, Kedwards and Lawrence, 1991).
Ask the patient to place the foot inside the Goretex bag.	To encourage co-operation of the patient and to apply the bag over the foot (Martin, French and Theakstone, 1990).Goretex bags offer a means of reducing the amount of accumulation of exudate and foot maceration, (Terrill, Kedwards and Lawrence, 1991).
Ensure the patient has enough room to spread the toes.	To allow for adequate movement inside the bag.
Gather the bag at the ankle and secure over the gauze by pulling the cord and tying in a bow or with a crepe bandage and adhesive tape.	To secure the bag in place — cords allow for the bag to be secured on the ankle and minimise the use of extra bandages. Tape is preferable to pins for the safety of the patient.
Apply splint(s) over the bag if required, on advice of medical staff and/or physiotherapist.	To allow for correct positioning of the foot and to minimise the risk of foot drop (Terrill, Kedwards and Lawrence, 1991).
Elevate the foot on pillows, avoid leg dangling and weight bearing.	To relieve venous congestion and minimise the collection of oedema (Sykes and Bailey, 1975).
Record in the appropriate documentation.	To maintain an accurate record.
Repeat the procedure on a daily basis or more often if required.	To allow for continual wound assessment and evaluation of treatment. For the comfort of the patient.
Throughout the day encourage active and passive exercises of the ankle and toes, involving a physiotherapist, as required.	Exercise maintains joint mobility and strengthens muscle tone (Martin, French and Theakstone, 1990). Advice can be given to patients on an exercise regime.

4. Procedure for applying a dressing to the foot

Dressings to the foot should be changed every 1–2 days. The aims of treatment are to minimise infection, remove dead tissue, provide a moist environment for wound healing and reduce swelling.

During treatment it is important to maintain a team approach with the physiotherapist and occupational therapist. Functional ability of the foot/ankle should be maximised by exercising frequently and applying splints where appropriate. The advantage of using dressings as opposed to bags is that the patient can mobilise safely without slipping on the cream and exudate inside the bag.

See sections 1–5 in Chapter 1 on advice on procedures.

Equipment

Trolley
Sterile dressing pack
Sterile scissors
1 pair of sterile gloves
2 pairs of unsterile gloves
Sachet of saline and alcohol swab
Paraffin gauze
Sterile towel
Sterile gauze swabs (large)
Sterile gauze swabs (small)
Crepe bandage and adhesive tape
Patient's prescription chart
Antibacterial cream (Silver Sulphadiazine) (optional)
Disposal bag
PVC (cling film)
Hand bath/bowl
Povidone Iodine aqueous solution 10% (optional)
Towel (optional)
Bacteriological wound swab (optional)

Action	Rationale
Administer analgesia as prescribed 30 minutes prior to commencing the procedure.	To minimise pain and discomfort for the patient.
Remove pillows from under the feet and ensure patient is in a comfortable position.	For the comfort of the patient.
Prepare the foot bath/bowl(s).	To ensure the foot bath is ready for use as soon as the dressings are removed.
– Fill three-quarters of the bath or bowl with warm water.	

Action	Rationale
– As an option add measured amount of Povidone Iodine aqueous solution 10% to the water and mix.	Povidone Iodine is an antibacterial solution effective in cleaning burn wounds (Brennan and Leaper, 1985). It is non irritant and has been used successfully for the treatment of burns (Wynn Williams and Montalliv, 1965; Cesany, 1977; de Kocke and van der Merwe, 1987).
Apply unsterile gloves.	For the protection of the nurse against body fluids and to minimise the risk of cross infection.
Remove existing dressing (leaving any gauze that is adherent) and discard in the disposal bag.	To minimise the risk of additional trauma caused by removing dressings that are adherent.
Remove gloves and wash hands.	To minimise the risk of cross infection.
If the wound appears red, inflamed, smells, or is oozing purulent discharge take a bacteriological wound swab for culture and sensitivity. Label and send to the microbiology laboratory.	To detect early signs of infection that may delay healing.
Gently lower the foot into the bath/bowl(s) and allow to soak.	Use of a foot bath will allow adherent dressings to be soaked off, minimise pain and assist with wound cleansing.
Apply unsterile gloves and using gauze swabs gently wipe over the foot and in between the toes.	Cleansing will facilitate the removal of old cream, dead skin, etc.
Encourage the patient to perform ankle exercises whilst immersing the foot in the bath.	Exercising is easier without restrictive dressings and allows free movement.
Remove foot and dry gently with gauze or a soft towel.	
Cover the foot with PVC (cling film).	To act as a temporary dressing while the contents of the foot bath are disposed of.
	To allow time for wound assessment by medical staff (if required) (Lendrum and Bowden Jones, 1976; Davies, 1983; Wilson and French, 1987; Milner, 1988).
Remove the foot bath/bowl(s) and contents away from the patient.	To remove dirty water and to minimise the risk of spillage.

Action	Rationale
Empty the contents of the bath/bowl(s) down the sluice/toilet.	To minimise the risk of cross infection.
Wash out the bath/bowl(s) with hot soapy water. Rinse and dry thoroughly and return to the appropriate storage area.	To minimise the risk of cross infection.
Remove gloves and wash hands.	To minimise the risk of cross infection.
Apply sterile gloves and place foot on the sterile towel.	To maintain asepsis.
If any exudate is present, moisten the gauze swabs with saline and, using the gloved hand, gently wipe over the skin and in between the toes.	To remove any exudate, scabs or loose skin.
Using sterile scissors burst and deroof any blisters.	Blisters are burst as they may restrict movement and cause discomfort for the patient. Also, blister fluid retards healing by impairing local immunity (Rockwell and Ehrlich, 1990; Anon, 1990). Deroofing the skin removes any dead skin that may harbour micro-organisms (Lawrence, 1989) and enables the nurse to assess the depth of the wound.
Using forceps, lift up any slough or loose dead tissue and using the sterile scissors cut as close to the skin as possible.	Slough and/or dead tissue may provide a focus for micro-organisms (Lawrence, 1989).
Apply a layer of antibacterial cream, e.g. Silver Sulphadiazine cream directly to the burn areas. **N.B. With burns to the toes, treat and apply dressings to each one separately.**	Seperate dressing to the toes prevents adherence of one wound surface to another which may cause webbing. May also facilitate easier movement. Silver Sulphadiazine cream is an antibacterial agent effective in the treatment of burns. (Sykes and Bailey, 1975; Hoffman, 1984).
Cover with 2–3 layers of paraffin gauze and gauze swabs (small sizes are available for use on toes) and Gamgee if excess exudate is expected.	Paraffin gauze is a bleached cotton gauze impregnated with Vaseline — it provides a non stick dressing and a moist environment for wound healing (Thomas, 1994). Gamgee is a bleached absorbent wool which is used to absorb exudate.
Avoid wrapping the paraffin gauze and gauze swabs circumferentially around the toes.	As oedema forms or drainage saturates the gauze and dries, constriction may result and the circulation may become impaired.

Action	Rationale
Apply crepe bandage occluding the toes (if necessary) and secure with adhesive tape at the ankle.	To secure dressings in place. Tape is preferable to pins for the safety of the patient.
Apply splint(s) over the dressings if required.	To allow for correct positioning of the foot and to minimise the risk of foot drop.
Elevate the foot on pillows, avoid leg dangling and weight bearing unless instructed by medical staff to encourage mobilisation.	To relieve venous congestion and minimise the collection of oedema (Sykes and Bailey, 1975).
Record in the appropriate documentation	To maintain an accurate record.
Repeat the procedure every 1–2 days or more often as directed by medical staff.	To allow for continual wound assessment and evaluation of treatment. Twice daily dressings may be required if wounds are infected, leaking or require intense physiotherapy.
Throughout the day encourage active and passive exercises of the ankle and toes.	Exercise maintains joint mobility and strengthens muscle tone.

References

Anon (1990) Should burn blisters be burst? Emergency Medicine 22 (1): 57–9.

Bailey BN, Desai SN (1973) An approach to the treatment of hand burns. Injury 4: 335.

Brennan SS, Leaper DJ (1985) The effects of antiseptics on the healing wound. British Journal of Surgery 72: 708–82.

Cesany P (1977) Clinical experience with povidone iodine (Betadine) in the treatment of burns and as an adjunct in plastic surgery. Pharmatherapeutica. 1: 514.

Davies JLW (1983) Synthetic materials for covering burn wounds. Progress towards perfection. Part I Short-term dressing material. Burns Journal 10: 94.

de Kocke M, van der Merwe AE (1987) A study to assess the effects of a new Betadine cream formulation compared to a standard topical treatment regimen for burns. Burns Journal. 13 (1): 69–74.

Fox CL (1968) Silver sulphadiazine — a new topical therapy for pseudomonas in burns. Archives of surgery 96: 18.

Garnes AL (1959) Clinical evaluation of povidone iodine in surgical practice. American Journal of Surgery 97: 49.

Hoffman S (1984) Silver sulphadiazine cream: an antibacterial agent for topical use in burns: A review of literature. Scandinavian Journal of Plastic and Reconstructive Surgery 18: 18, 119.

Kemble JV, Lamb BE (1987) Practical Burns Management. London: Hodder and Stoughton.

Konop DJ (1991) General local treatment. In Trofino RB (Ed) Nursing Care of the Burn-Injured Patient Philadelphia: FA Davies Company. pp 55–6.

Lawrence JC (1989) Management of burns. The Dressing Times 2 (3): 1–4.

Lendrum J, Bowden-Jones E (1976) A new dressing for burns. Enclosure in a plasticised polyvinylchloride sheet. Burns Journal 3 (2): 86.

Lowbury ELJ, Jackson DM, Ricketts CR et al., (1971) Topical chemoprophylaxis for burns. Trials of creams containing silver sulphadiazine and trimethoprim. Injury 3: 18.

Martin DL, French GWG, Theakstone J (1990) The use of semi-permeable membranes for wound management. British Journal of Plastic Surgery 43: 55–60.

Martin MT (1991) Burns of the Hands and Feet. In Trofino RB (Ed) Nursing Care of the Burn-Injured Patient Philadelphia: FA Davies Company. pp 212–21.

Milner RH (1988) Plasticised polyvinylchloride film as primary burns dressing — A microbiological study. Burns Journal 14 (1): 62–5.

Muddiman R (1989) A new concept in hand burn dressings. Nursing Standard (Special Supplement) September pp 23: 1–3.

Pegg SP (1982) The role of drugs in management of burns. Drugs 24: 256.

Reid WH (1974) Care of the burned hand. Hand 6: 163.

Richards RME, Mahlangu GN (1981) Therapy for burn wound infection. Journal of Clinical Hospital Pharmacy 6: 233.

Rockwell C, Ehrlich HP (1990) Should burn blisters be burst? Journal of Burn Care and Rehabilitation 11: 93.

Slater RM, Hughes NC (1971) A simplified method of treating burns of the hands. British Journal of Plastic Surgery. 24: 296–300.

Stanford W, Rappole BW, Fox CL (1969) Clinical experience with silver sulphadiazine. Journal of Trauma 9: 377.

Sykes PJ, Bailey BN (1975) Treatment of hand burns with occlusive bags: A comparison of three methods. Burns Journal 2: 163.

Terrill PJ, Kedwards SM, Lawrence JC (1991) The use of Goretex bags for hand burns. Burns Journal 17 (2): 161–5.

Thomas S (1994) Jelonet. In Thomas S (Ed) Handbook of Wound Dressings. London: MacMillan. pp 98–9.

Van Saene JJM, Trooster JFG, Meulenhoff AMC, Lerk CF (1987) Release and antimicrobial activity of silver sulphadiazine from different creams. Burns Journal 13 (2): 123–30.

Wilson G, French G (1987) Plasticised polyvinylchloride as a temporary dressing for burns. British Medical Journal 294: 556–7.

Wilson GR, Fowler CA, Housden PL (1987) A new burn area assessment chart. Burns Journal 13 (5): 401–5.

Wilson J (1992) Theory and practice of isolation nursing. Nursing Standard 1 (18): 30–1.

Wynn-Williams D, Montalliv G (1965) The effects of povidone iodine in the treatment of burns and traumatic losses of skin. Journal of Plastic Surgery 18: 146.

Further reading

Gamgee JS (1880) Absorbent and medical surgical dressings. Lancet 57 127.

Chapter 11
Care of patient with perineal burns

A perineal burn is a physically and emotionally traumatic injury. Acute pain, anxiety and embarrassment are all-important considerations in nursing care. The majority of burns to the perineal area are caused by flame, contact burns, scalds, chemicals and, in some cases, are secondary to abuse, neglect and/or assault (Balakrishnan et al., 1995).

Children may fall into the category of victims of abuse due to unsuccessful toilet training or may suffer immersion scalds. Spouse abuse is suspected when the patient is reluctant or refuses to discuss how the accident happened. Elderly abuse/neglect is often due to individuals left unattended or unsupervised in a bath or who have bladder and bowel problems.

Burns to the perineum are serious injuries not only because of their delicate location but also because they may pose problems related to treatment and wound healing. Perineal burns may result in scarring and functional impairment and tend to increase the patient's anxieties because of the changes in body image and the nature of the pain and discomfort that is experienced due to the sensitive areas involved (Konop, 1991).

The position of perineal burns differs according to gender. In females perineal burns involve the pubis and inner thighs. The vulva is rarely involved: due to its anatomical position it is generally protected from direct burn trauma. However, swelling of the labia may occur due to oedema formation. In males the genitalia are exposed, less protected and more likely to be affected by direct trauma. Groin and/or thighs may be involved and gross oedema of the penis and scrotum usually occurs as a result of burns to the perineal area. This added complication causes discomfort and embarrassment to the patient. Care must be taken to provide adequate scrotal support during this stage.

In both sexes, oedema formation in the genitals may cause obstruction of the urethra and the patient may be unable to pass urine. Insertion of a urinary catheter keeps the urethra patent, allows drainage of urine and avoids contamination of wounds with urine in the early stages. In extreme cases a suprapubic catheter may need to be inserted.

Perineal burns are usually painful, the severity will be influenced by the depth and the percentage body surface area involved. Superficial and partial thickness burns are very sensitive due to exposure of nerve endings and, even with full thickness burns there may be some areas of partial thickness injury so these will be equally painful. In order to minimise the pain and discomfort administer analgesia at regular intervals as prescribed on the patient's prescription chart and monitor its effectiveness.

In extensive injuries to the buttocks, thighs and perineum, the use of an air fluidised bed is advocated to lessen discomfort associated with lying and sitting.

In general, management of burns to the perineum or genital area is aimed at minimising pain and discomfort, paying attention to cleanliness and personal hygiene, preventing infection and promoting healing.

It is imperative that patients with perineal burns receive frequent and extensive explanations of treatment throughout, with the provision of counselling and emotional support as required.

1. Procedure for the care of a patient with perineal burns on admission to the Burns Unit

It is important that perineal burns are evaluated and treated by both medical and nursing staff who are adequately trained in burn care. Therefore, admitting the patient to a Burns Unit is both appropriate and necessary.

On admission, a detailed history relating to the injury is required. Circumstances and events must be investigated and reported if necessary as abuse is frequently a cause of perineal burns.

See sections 1–3 in Chapter 1 for advice on procedures.

Equipment

    Tray/trolley
    Sterile gloves
    Unsterile gloves
    Sterile towel
    Burns assessment chart
    Patient's prescription card
    Light source

Action	Rationale
On admission to the Burns Unit transfer the patient into a single room and nurse in protective isolation.	To minimise the risk of cross infection. To maintain privacy in nursing the burn area exposed in some instances.
Maintain privacy and dignity for the patient at *all* times.	To reduce embarrassment and anxiety during the procedure.

Action	Rationale
Obtain a detailed history of the injury, e.g. cause and duration of contact. Note any signs of the possibility of abuse, e.g. patient withdrawn, unwilling to discuss injury.	To assist in ascertaining the severity of the injury. Circumstances and events surrounding the injury should be investigated as abuse is a frequent cause (Konop, 1991).
– If a chemical injury note the type, duration of contact and any first aid treatment undertaken.	Inadequate first aid treatment may indicate a need to irrigate the burn injured area further to dilute the chemical and minimise further damage to the tissues (Konop, 1991).
N.B. Contact the poison centre if chemical unknown.	To determine appropriate antidote.
Ask the patient if he or she has any pain, noting quality and intensity. Administer analgesia as prescribed by the medical staff on the patient's prescription chart.	Perineal burns are usually very sensitive (Konop, 1991).
Assist the patient into a comfortable position and ensure an adequate light source before commencing an examination of the perineal area.	To facilitate easier inspection of the perineum.
Apply sterile gloves and place the sterile towel under the patient's buttocks.	To maintain asepsis.
Perform a physical inspection of the perineal area.	
Observe for:	
– Areas of perineum/genitalia involved.	To determine the extent of the percentage body surface area involved (Wilson, Fowler and Housden, 1987).
– Presence of any skin loss.	The anatomy of the perineum/genitalia may allow some creases/skinfolds to be spared (Konop, 1991).
– Lacerations/abrasions.	
– Oedema	Oedema formation may cause obstruction of the urethra.
Insert a urinary catheter if:	
– Swelling around the urethra is observed. or	To avoid obstruction of urine flow due to swelling.
– Patient complains of pain on voiding urine. or	To minimise the risk of the patient developing retention from refusal to pass urine.
– Patient has no bladder control. (Refer to sections 4 and 5 below on the procedure for male/female catheterisation.)	Continual contact of the wounds with urine may cause excoriation and further damage to tissue.

Action	Rationale
Monitor and record urine output.	Urine output indicates adequacy of fluid replacement following a burn injury and indicates patency of catheter.
Ensure careful attention to personal cleanliness around the perineal/genital areas.	To minimise contamination and infection (Konop, 1991).
Record history and physical examination on the appropriate assessment charts and in the appropriate documentation.	To maintain an accurate record.
Treat the areas exposed discretely by maintaining protective isolation throughout and apply topical anti-bacterial creams 4-6 hourly. or – Apply topical antibacterial creams, with minimal non constricting dressings and renew 4–6 hourly or after voiding urine or defaecation.	To minimise the risk of cross infection (Konop, 1991). To minimise infection and for the comfort of the patient.

2. Procedure for the care of burns to the perineum

The management of burns to the perineum or genital area is aimed at minimising infection and promoting healing (Peck et al., 1990).

The use of frequent cleansing and the application of topical antibacterial creams is advocated using a conservative approach. Surgical intervention is not recommended in the first instance as the skin in this area has many folds and creases and in a burn injury many areas may be spared thus allowing the wound to heal (Konop, 1991).

A urinary catheter may be inserted on admission to assist with urinary drainage therefore catheter care is an important aspect of routine care. (Refer to sections 4 and 5 on the procedure for male/female catheterisation.)

See sections 1–5 in Chapter 1 for advice on procedures.

Equipment

Trolley
Sterile dressing pack
Sterile scissors
1 pair of unsterile gloves
1 pair of sterile gloves
Sterile/protective field
Sachets of normal saline and alcohol swab
Paraffin gauze
Antibacterial cream (Silver Sulphadiazine)

Gamgee
Moisturising cream/lubricating gel
Bacteriological wound swab (optional)
Universal container (optional)
Disposal bag
Patient's prescription chart

Action	Rationale
Isolate the patient in a single room if the burns are discretely exposed and the application of dressings are inappropriate.	Protective isolation minimises the risk of cross infection (Konop, 1991).
Administer analgesia as prescribed on the patient's prescription chart.	To minimise pain and discomfort for the patient.
Apply unsterile gloves, remove dressing and discard in disposal bag.	To protect the nurse from body fluids and to minimise the risk of cross infection.
Remove gloves and wash hands.	To minimise the risk of cross infection.
Observe the wound for redness, swelling, odour and the presence of pus or discharge.	To detect signs of infection.
If any evidence of infection take a bacteriological wound swab, label and send to the microbiology laboratory for culture and sensitivity.	To detect any infection which may delay healing or require treatment.
Clip away any hair on or near the burn areas (if required).	Hair is a medium for bacterial growth, removal of hair minimises the risk of infection (Konop, 1991).
Apply sterile gloves and position the sterile protective field under the patient's perineum.	To minimise the risk of cross infection.
Moisten the gauze swabs with saline.	
Using the gauze gently clean the perineum and/or genital area.	To remove any dead tissue and/or exudate (Peck et al., 1990).
Using the sterile scissors, burst any blisters and expel the fluid but avoid totally deroofing the blisters.	Deroofing blisters in this sensitive area will cause pain due to nerve endings being exposed.
Using forceps, gently lift up any loose skin or slough and using the sterile scissors cut off as close to the skin as possible.	Dead skin and/or slough can be a focus for bacterial growth (Lawrence, 1989).
Using more moistened gauze swabs clean the perineal/genital area including the area around the urinary catheter (if appropriate).	To minimise the risk of urinary tract infections.

Action	Rationale
Apply a thin layer of Silver Sulphadiazine — an antibacterial cream — onto the burn areas.	Silver Sulphadiazine cream is an antimicrobial agent effective in the treatment of burns. To minimise infection (Hamilton-Miller, Shah and Smith, 1991).
Cover with double layers of paraffin gauze (if both vulva and labia are involved, separate the surfaces with layers of paraffin gauze).	Paraffin gauze is a bleached cotton gauze impregnated with soft paraffin and is effective as a non-stick dressing (Thomas, 1994). Separation of the surfaces minimises the risk of contractures and/or webbing. If adjacent burn surfaces are not separated they can adhere to each other.
Cover with layers of sterile gauze and Gamgee (if required).	To absorb excess exudate (Gamgee, 1980) and to provide a temporary occlusive dressing.
Secure in place with a nappy (if toddler) or patient's own underwear.	For the comfort of the patient and to prevent the dressing from becoming displaced.
If the use of dressings is inappropriate, treat the wounds exposed. Sit the patient on a pad of paraffin gauze and Gamgee and insert a bed cradle over the bed.	To minimise pain and discomfort while the patient is sitting or lying and to minimise cross infection. A bed cradle will keep top bed linen away from the perineum. To maintain dignity.
If the patient has a urinary catheter *in situ*: – Position catheter and drainage tubing appropriately whilst in bed. – Secure tubing to the patient's leg if mobilising.	To facilitate the flow of urine into the drainage tube and to minimise pain and discomfort for the patient caused by poor positioning or excess tension on the tubing.
In male patients observe for the presence of scrotal oedema. If evident: – Elevate scrotum on Gamgee or a soft towel whilst lying in bed.	Elevation will assist with reducing pain and oedema.
– Apply a scrotal support if mobilising.	A scrotal support will minimise discomfort while mobilising.
Explain to the patient the importance of not touching the dressings and to avoid rubbing or scratching the perineal/genital area.	To minimise the risk of cross infection. Rubbing and/or scratching will cause friction that may destroy new epithelial cells and delay healing (McDougall et al., 1979).
If the patient has an indwelling urinary catheter, repeat the procedure twice daily.	For the comfort of the patient.

Action	Rationale
If the patient does not have a urinary catheter, repeat the procedure each time urine is passed or after a bowel movement. Monitor urine output and frequency of bowel actions.	Contamination of the wounds from urine or faeces may cause skin irritation, infection, or delay wound healing (Konop, 1991; Renz and Sherman, 1993). Pain may cause the patient to be reluctant to pass urine or open the bowels causing retention and/or constipation.
Monitor and record the patient's temperature 4 hourly. If the temperature rises above 38.5° C:	
— Take a bacteriological wound swab (at the next dressing change) for culture and sensitivity. Label and send to the microbiology laboratory.	To detect any infection which may require treatment.
— Collect a specimen of urine (CSU or MSU) for culture and sensitivity. Empty into universal container, label and send to the microbiology laboratory.	To detect a urinary tract infection which may occur as a result of burns to the perineum or an indwelling urinary catheter.
Apply moisturising/lubricating agents to the perineal/genital area as healing progresses.	Healed skin becomes more sensitive, dry and itchy and may cause discomfort for the patient.
Assess the wound on a daily basis and record in the appropriate documentation.	To observe wound healing and to monitor and record appropriateness of treatment.

3. Care of a patient requiring an in-dwelling urethral catheter

Having decided that urethral catheterisation is in the best interest of the patient, the following criteria should be considered when selecting the catheter and drainage system:

1. Catheter size
2. Balloon size
3. Material of the catheter
4. Drainage bag

Catheter size

The rule is "small is best" i.e. 12 (fg) or possibly 14 (fg) if there is debris present (Crummey, 1989).

Females should be offered the appropriate female length (much shorter) catheter if mobile. If a male length catheter is used, pooling of urine will occur in the loop of the catheter that is not needed. The extra length may also catch on clothing, etc. causing trauma through tension.

Larger size catheters have been found to be associated with leakage of urine, bypassing around the catheter and causing the patient discomfort (Roe, 1986;

Kennedy and Brocklehurst, 1982). This is because the shape of the urethra is elliptical and if a larger diameter catheter is used, it becomes distended, creating spaces either side of the catheter for leakage of urine.

Balloon size

Once again, small is best, i.e. 10 ml. A larger balloon causes a larger residual volume of urine.

Leakage of urine has been attributed not only to the size of the catheter but also to the size of the balloon. It has been found that larger balloons cause irritation of the mucosa and trigone, which leads to spasm and hence bypassing (Blannin and Hobden, 1980).

It should also be noted that if a larger balloon is partially inflated, it leans over to one side, which may also cause irritation and trauma to the bladder wall.

Material of the catheter

According to Sutton (1992) the probable period of time the patient needs to be catheterised, and the patient's comfort are important factors to consider.

Catheters made of latex are said by manufacturers to be suitable for only short-term use, up to 21 days, as they tend to become encrusted more quickly. However, some patients find them more comfortable because they are softer. All silicone catheters are said to be for long-term use — anything from 21 days to 3 months. Silicone is the most inert substance available and therefore is less prone to encrustation. However, it is less flexible than latex, and is about three times more expensive. Hydrogel-coated catheters are the latest addition to the range of materials available. The limited research available so far would suggest that the unique quality of the coating is beneficial to the patient and they can therefore be recommended for long-term use, i.e. 3 months.

Drainage bag

Selection of the drainage system depends on the individual patient.

The first criteria is that the catheter and drainage bag should be disconnected as infrequently as possible. Therefore, a leg drainage bag should be used if the patient is out of bed. There are a range of capacities available, with long or short inlet tubes. For example, a man may prefer a long inlet tube, so that he can wear the bag strapped to his calf. A woman would probably find a short tube, with a smaller capacity bag more discreet, and may wear it in a suitable pair of pants.

At night, a 2 litre drainable drainage bag should be attached to the bottom of the leg bag with the connecting tap left open. The 2 litre bag is then emptied and discarded next morning. The leg bag may stay *in situ* for up to one week.

In summary, the selection of the catheter and drainage bag should be made carefully according to the individual patient's needs.

4. Procedure for male catheterisation

Initial catheterisation must be carried out by the medical staff. Recatheterisation may be undertaken by the medical staff or a nurse trained to carry out this procedure.

See sections 1– 5 in Chapter I, for advice on procedures and sharps policy.

Equipment

Trolley
Sterile catheterisation pack
2 pairs of sterile gloves
Sterile tube of local anaesthetic gel (with nozzle)
Sachet of saline and alcohol swab
2 catheters (of appropriate size and material)
10 ml sterile syringe and needle
10 ml ampoule of sterile water
Drainage bag
Straps or stand
Non-allergic tape
Sharps box

Action	Rationale
Apply sterile gloves, open sterile pack and prepare equipment.	To maintain asepsis (Wright, 1988).
Attach sterile nozzle to tube of local anaesthetic gel.	To maintain sterility of local anaesthetic gel (if required).
Draw up 5–10 ml of water into the syringe (depending on catheter balloon capacity).	
Retract the patient's foreskin (if possible) and clean the glans with saline.	To remove smegma (desquamated epithelial cells found chiefly under the foreskin) and to minimise the risk of infection.
Insert the local anaesthetic gel into the urethra until it begins to ooze back out.	To maximise the effects of the local anaesthetic.
Wait for 2–3 minutes.	This allows the optimum effect of the local anaesthetic to be achieved.
Remove first pair of sterile gloves. Wash hands and apply second pair of sterile gloves.	To minimise the risk of cross infection.
Retract the foreskin (if necessary). Hold the penis upright and insert the catheter slowly. If resistance is felt stop for a short time, and ask the patient to cough or bear down.	To ensure a straight pathway for catheter insertion. Resistance may be felt at the external sphincter (5–20 cm) after insertion, asking the patient to cough may overcome this (Pomfret, 1993) and this may relax the sphincters.

Action	Rationale
Continue to insert the catheter until urine comes out. Relax the foreskin.	To ascertain the position of the catheter in the bladder.
N.B. If no urine drains when the full length of the catheter has been inserted then wait for 5 minutes to see if any drainage occurs. If not seek medical advice.	The end of the catheter may be curled up in the prostatic bed.
(Do not inflate the balloon.)	Inflation may result in trauma if the catheter is not in the bladder.
When urine is draining, place the end of the catheter in a sterile receiver and inflate the balloon to the specified amount using the syringe containing sterile water.	To inflate the balloon and to ensure the catheter remains *in situ.*
Connect the catheter to the drainage bag.	To establish a closed sterile circuit.
Using hypo-allergenic tape anchor the catheter to the inner aspect of the thigh allowing sufficient free tubing to allow for an erection.	To prevent unnecessary trauma to the urethra, which may cause discomfort and increase the risk of infection (Lowthian, 1988; Slade and Gillespie, 1985).
Record in the appropriate nursing documentation.	To maintain an accurate record.

5. Procedure for female catheterisation

Catheterisation may be carried out by the medical staff or a nurse trained to carry out this procedure.

See sections 1–5 in Chapter 1 for advice on procedures and sharps policy.

Equipment

Trolley
Sterile catheterisation pack
2 pairs of sterile gloves
Sterile tube of local anaesthetic gel (with nozzle)
Sachet of saline and alcohol swabs
2 catheters (of appropriate size and material)
10 ml sterile syringe and needle
10 ml ampoule of sterile water
Sterile towel
Drainage bag
Straps or stand
Non-allergic tape

Action	Rationale
Position patient to allow access to the vulval area in whatever manner is most comfortable and appropriate for the patient.	To maintain patient comfort.
Apply sterile gloves, open sterile pack and prepare equipment.	To maintain asepsis.
Position the sterile towel under the patient's buttocks and thighs.	To maintain asepsis.
Draw up 5–10 ml of water into the syringe depending on the catheter balloon capacity.	
Clean the vulval area from the pubic bone to the perineal area using gauze swabs soaked in saline, using each swab once only. Clean each side, then down the middle.	To prevent introducing infection into the urinary tract.
Insert the local anaesthetic gel into the urethra.	To minimise discomfort for the patient during the procedure and to dilate the urethra, facilitating easier less painful passage of the catheter.
Wait for 3–4 minutes.	Optimum time for gel to take effect (De-Courey-Ireland, 1993).
Remove gloves, wash hands and apply second pair of sterile gloves.	To minimise the risk of cross infection.
Place the catheter, retained in its inner wrap in the receiver and place close to the patient on the sterile field.	To maintain asepsis and to allow ease of access to the catheter.
Separate the labia, identify the urethral orifice and insert the catheter until urine flows out. (If the catheter is accidentally inserted into the vagina, leave it there whilst inserting a new one into the urethra.)	Prevents misplacement of the catheter a second time.
Leaving the catheter draining into the receiver, inflate the balloon to the specified amount using the syringe and sterile water as previously prepared.	Inflating the balloon ensures the catheter remains *in situ*.
Attach the catheter to the appropriate drainage bag.	To establish a closed circuit.
Using hypo-allergenic tape anchor the catheter to the inner aspect of the thigh allowing for normal body movement.	To prevent trauma to the urethra (Lowthian, 1988) and to minimise infection (Slade and Gillespie, 1985).
Record in the appropriate nursing documentation.	To maintain an accurate record.

6. Procedure for meatal cleansing and general care of the catheterised patient

Organisms are known to pass from the perineum to the bladder, particularly under water. Therefore, showers are preferable to baths for catheterised patients. Normal personal hygiene would dictate a shower or bed bath daily, and other cleansing of the meatus should be carried out only if necessary to keep the patient comfortable. Soap and water plus single use cloth/wipe should be used and disposable gloves worn (Wright, 1989). Because organisms are known to travel back to the bladder through air bubbles, the drainage bag must be positioned well below the level of the patient's bladder at all times to prevent back flow of both air and urine. The drainage tubing of the bag should be clamped, not the catheter (Lowthian, 1988) and the bag left attached to maintain the closed system and prevent back flow (Roe, 1990). See Figure 11.1 for potential sites for bacteria to enter into the closed urinary drainage system. Any manipulation of the catheter should be kept to a minimum. An aseptic technique should be used to reduce the risk of introducing infection into the system (Lowthian, 1988). Urine must be allowed to drain freely with no kinks or tension at any point in the system

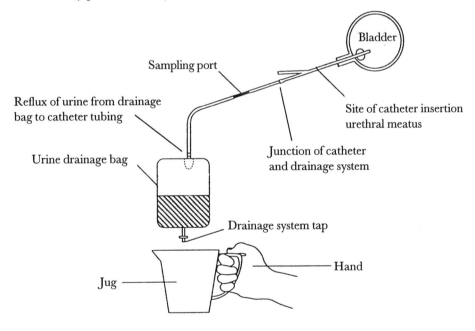

Figure 11.1 *Potential sites for bacteria to enter into a closed urinary drainage system.*

References

Balakrishnan C, Imel LL, Bandy AT, Prasad JK (1995) Perineal burns secondary to spouse abuse. Journal of the International Society for Burn Injuries 21 (1): 34–5.

Blannin JP, Hobden J (1980) The catheter of choice. Nursing Times 76: 2020–93.

Crummey V (1989) Ignorance can hurt. Nursing Times. 85 (21): 65–70.

De-Courey-Ireland A (1993) An issue of sensitivity-use of analgesic gel in catheterising women. Professional Nurse. 8 (11): 738–42.

Gamgee JS (1880) Absorbent and medical surgical dressings, Lancet. 57: 127.

Hamilton-Muller JMT, Shah S, Smith C (1993) Silver sulphadiazine a comprehensive *in vitro* reassessment Chemotherapy 39: 405–9.

Kennedy AP, Brocklehurst JC (1982) The nursing management of patients with long-term indwelling catheters. Journal of Advanced Nursing. 7: 411–17.

Konop DJ (1991) Perineal burns. In Trofino RB (Ed) Nursing Care of the Burn-Injured Patient Philadelphia: EA Davis Company. pp 202–11.

Lawrence JC (1989) Management of burns. The Dressing Times 2 (3): 1–4.

Lowthian P (1988) Steps to combat infection. Nursing Times 84 (12): 64–6.

McDougall WS et al. (1979) The thermally injured perineum. Journal of Urology 121 (3): 320.

Peck MD, Boileau MA, Grube BJ, Heimbach DM (1990) The management of burns to the perineum and genitals. Journal of Burn Care and Rehabilitation. 11: 54–6.

Pomfret P (1993) Men only. Male catheterisation. Nursing Times. 89 (8): 55–8.

Renz BM, Sherman R (1993) Exposure of buttock burn wounds to stool in scald abuse infants and children — stool staining of eschar and burn wound sepsis. American Surgeon 59: 379–83.

Roe BH (1986) Patients perception of their catheters and study of urine drainage system. University of Manchester: MCS Thesis.

Roe BH (1990) Do we need to clamp catheters? Nursing Times 86 (43): 31–3.

Slade N, Gillespie WA (1985) The urinary tract and the catheter — infection and other problems. Chichester: Wiley.

Sutton T (1992) Material benefits. Nursing Times. 88 (31): 61–2.

Thomas S (1994) Jelonet. In Thomas S (Ed) Handbook of Wound Dressings. London: MacMillan. pp 98–9.

Wilson GR, Fowler CA, Housden PL (1987) A new burn area assessment chart. Burns Journal 13 (5): 401–5.

Wright E (1988) Minimising the risk of UTI. Professional Nurse. 4: 63–7.

Wright E (1989) Teaching patients to cope with catheters at home. Professional Nurse. 14: 191–2.

Further Reading

Furnas DW, McCrow JB (1980) Resurfacing the genital area. Clinical Plastic Surgery .17 (2): 235.

Chapter 12
Care of a patient with an electrical burn injury

High voltage electrical injuries are well described in the literature (Baxter, 1970; Burke, Quinby and Bordoc, 1977; Christiensen et al., 1980; Nichter et al., 1984; Reiche and Kay, 1985; Wang et al., 1985; Shen, Chang and Wang, 1990; Koller, 1991). However, reports on low voltage burns are not as evident (Gordon, Reid and Awaad, 1986).

According to Lee and Kolodney (1987 a,b) and Gordon, Reid and Awaad (1986) electricity can cause injury to the body in three ways. Firstly the electrical energy may be converted to light causing damage to the eye. Secondly, the passage of an electrical current through the body can effect the brain and the heart. Thirdly, the injury may be a result of the conversion of electrical energy to heat.

In general terms, there are three types of electrical burn injuries (Trofino and Orr, 1991).

1. Thermal body surface burns as a result of ignition of clothing from heat or flames produced by an electrical spark.
2. Severe deep injuries associated with high voltage current arcing onto the skin.
3. Direct contact of the body with an electrical source, e.g. a live wire enabling the current to travel through the tissue creating injuries to deeper areas producing entrance and exit wounds.

In an electrical burn injury the current (high or low voltage, direct or alternating) enters the body at the point of contact, travels along planes and structures of low resistance and exits through the earth contact (Kemble and Lamb, 1987). In the first instance only the entry and exit points will produce visible skin injury but the severity of electrical burns is affected by the:

1. Type and voltage of the circuit.
2. Amperage of the current.
3. Resistance of the body.
4. Pathway of the current.
5. Duration of contact (Trofino and Orr, 1991).

The extent of damage is a result of:

1. Heat caused by the current travelling through the tissues.
2. Damage to blood vessels resulting in thrombosis of blood vessels and necrosis.
3. Alterations to the electrical conductivity of the heart and nerves.
4. Tetanic muscle contractions.
5. Strong spasmodic movement of the body causing spinal or limb fractures.
6. Thermal body surface area burns as a result of clothing catching fire (Kemble and Lamb, 1987).

As a result of the electrical burn injury many physiological changes may occur in the body:

1. Skin damage at the point of contact.
2. Internal destruction of blood vessels, nerves, muscles.
3. Paraesthesia or quadriplegia due to compression fractures of the vertebrae or disruption of blood supply to the spinal cord. Altered neurological status, e.g. confusion, convulsions, loss of consciousness, respiratory depression.
4. Cardiac irregularities, ventricular fibrillation.
5. Altered electrolyte balance, e.g. hypokalaemia.
6. Release of myoglobin into the circulatory system as a result of muscle damage.
7. Increased haemoglobinuria and haematuria from damaged tissue.
8. Acute tubular necrosis and renal failure.

Although the literature contains much information concerning the mechanisms of electrical injury (Lee, 1961; Lee and Kolodney, 1987a,b), the types of injury (Hanumadass et al., 1986; Koller, 1991) and the types of wounds (Holliman et al., 1982), management of such injuries remains a troublesome problem.

1. Procedure for the care of a patient following an electrical burn injury on admission to the Burns Unit

All patients admitted to the Burns Unit should be assessed immediately for vital organ function. In the UK the household voltage of 240 volts can cause ventricular fibrillation or respiratory paralysis (Lee, 1961; Sturim, 1971), and may result in death (Solem, Fisher and Strate, 1977; Sances et al., 1979; Arturson and Hedlund, 1984). Monitoring the cardiac rate and rhythm is very important as dysrhythmias may occur due to disruption of the cardiac cycle. An electrocardiogram should be obtained as soon as possible after the injury to assess possible cardiac abnormalities (Trofino and Orr, 1991), and continued for 24 hours.

Monitoring pulses on affected limbs proximal and distal to the entrance and exit wounds should also be a priority during the initial assessment.

Neurological assessments may indicate central nervous system involvement, with evidence of confusion, convulsions, loss of consciousness and respiratory depression.

See sections 1 and 2 in Chapter 1 for advice on procedures and sharps policy.

Equipment

Tray/trolley
Unsterile gloves
PVC (cling film)
Doppler machine (optional)
ECG monitor, leads and electrodes
Selection of sterile syringes, needles, blood specimen bottles
Tourniquet (of appropriate size)
Burns assessment chart
Nursing documentation chart
Patient's prescription chart
Sharps box

Action	Rationale
On admission of the patient to the Burns Unit, obtain a detailed history of the injury, e.g. cause, voltage of the current (if known), and duration of contact with the source.	To assist in ascertaining the severity of the injury. History allows for appropriate interventions to be performed (Trofino and Orr, 1991).
Determine if any first aid treatment was undertaken and the condition of the patient when rescued.	To assess whether appropriate interventions have been performed. To determine if cardiopulmonary resuscitation was required at the scene.
Prepare the ECG monitor: – Attach the electrodes to the chest. – Connect the leads and plug them into the monitor. – Switch on the monitor. – Observe and record the result over a 24-hour period.	Electrical burn injuries may cause cardiac arrhythmias. Monitoring of cardiac status is advised for 24 hours post electrical burn injury to assess cardiac damage (Kemble and Lamb, 1987; Trofino and Orr, 1991). Occasionally, patients may develop a myocardial infarction or arrhythmia that requires treatment (Butler and Grant, 1977; Solem, Fisher and Strate, 1977; Szabo and Ver, 1983; Arturson and Hedlund, 1984).
Ask the patient if they have any pain, noting quality and intensity. Administer analgesia as prescribed by the medical staff.	To minimise pain and discomfort for the patient.
Apply unsterile gloves.	To protect the nurse from body fluids and minimise the risk of cross infection.
Remove any jewellery, e.g. rings or bracelets circumferentially surrounding any extremities.	With the oedema formation that follows a burn injury, circumferential pressure may reduce perfusion and cause tissue damage.

Action	Rationale
Perform a physical inspection of the body.	To assess the extent of the injury.
Observe:	
– Integrity of the skin and note exposure of any underlying structures, e.g. tendons, joints, muscles.	
– Extent of skin loss.	To estimate the percentage body surface area burns (Wilson, Fowler and Housden, 1987). In some cases it may be valueless as the tissue destruction is both internal and external.
– Appearance of the skin, e.g. black, charred, ischaemic.	Determines the depth of tissue destruction.
– Presence of entry and exit wounds.	Determines direct contact of the body with an electrical source.
– Absent or diminishing pulses in the limbs. **N.B. The use of a Doppler machine may be advocated if pulses are difficult to palpate.**	Absent or weak pulses indicate that an escharotomy may be required to accommodate the swelling and permit blood flow to the extremities (Trofino and Orr, 1991).
– Appearance of the limbs, e.g. charred, contracted, absent.	May indicate a high voltage electrical burn (Trofino and Orr, 1991).
– Evidence of any fractures and/or dislocations of joints. Assist with positioning the patient for an X-ray (if required).	The patient may have sustained fractures and/or dislocations of joints from severe muscle contractures resulting from the injury. An X-ray will determine the extent of the injuries (Trofino and Orr, 1991).
When inspection is complete, apply a layer of PVC (cling film) over the burn wounds until they have been assessed by the medical staff	To provide a temporary non-stick dressing (Wilson and French, 1987) until the prescribed dressings are applied.
Assist the doctor with an escharotomy (see appropriate procedure) if required.	To allow for the expansion of the skin caused by the development of oedema, to allow unrestricted blood flow to the extremities and to preserve tissue which would otherwise become non-viable (Kemble and Lamb, 1987; Trofino and Orr, 1991).
Observe for any burns on the abdomen and instigate prompt treatment.	Burns on the abdomen may cause thrombosis of intestinal vessels which may lead to intestinal gangrene (Kemble and Lamb, 1987), infection, extensive necrosis and even death (Zhu, Yu, Wang and Zhoo, 1993).

Action	Rationale
Assist the doctor in obtaining a sample of blood for full blood count, urea and electrolytes.	As a result of an extensive electrical burn injury, altered electrolyte balance may occur, e.g. hypokalaemia.
Obtain a specimen of urine and test for colour, pH, specific gravity, blood, protein and urobilogen.	Damaged muscles release myoglobin into the urine which can lead to acute tubular necrosis and renal failure.
Monitor and record urine output on a fluid balance chart.	To monitor fluid balance and to detect early signs of renal complications (Trofino and Orr, 1991).
Record the history and physical examination in the appropriate documentation.	To maintain an accurate record.

2. Procedure for the care of electrical burns

The damage from an electrical current depends on the specific resistance of individual tissues and their sensitivity to heat damage. Bone has the greatest resistance to current flow and therefore generates most heat (Fried et al., 1991)

A patient who has sustained an electrical injury may present with many different injuries. Limbs may be contracted, immobile and charred. Entrance wounds from direct electrical contact are whitish-yellow in appearance and ischaemic whilst exit wounds are grey-white, black in the centre, and accompanied by complete tissue loss and exposed underlying structures (Trofino and Orr, 1991).

Low voltage electrical burn injuries usually appear as small puncture wounds. The extent of tissue destruction becomes more marked 3–5 days post injury so are treated initially with local dressings until the wounds are surgically debrided and the appropriate skin graft or flap is performed (Kemble and Lamb, 1987).

High voltage injuries are more severe and escharotomies may be required as oedema progresses. Removal of muscle and/or amputation of limbs may be advocated in extreme cases.

See sections 1–5 in Chapter 1 for advice on procedures.

Equipment

Trolley
Sterile dressing pack
Sterile scissors
Sachet of normal saline and alcohol swab
1 pair of unsterile gloves
1 pair of sterile gloves
Sterile gauze swabs
Paraffin gauze

Antibacterial cream (Silver Sulphadiazine)
Bandage (of appropriate size)
Bacteriological wound swab (optional)
Adhesive tape
Disposal bag
Patient's prescription chart

Action	Rationale
Administer prescribed analgesia approximately 30 minutes prior to commencing the procedure.	To minimise pain and discomfort for the patient.
Apply unsterile gloves. Remove existing dressing and discard into the disposal bag.	For the protection of the nurse against body fluids and to minimise the risk of cross infection.
Remove gloves and wash hands.	To minimise the risk of cross infection.
If any of the wounds appear red, inflamed, painful, malodorous or are oozing purulent discharge, take a bacteriological wound swab. Label and send to the microbiology laboratory for culture and sensitivity.	To detect any infection which may delay healing or require treatment.
Apply sterile gloves.	To maintain asepsis.
Moisten the sterile gauze with saline.	Moistened gauze will facilitate easy removal of exudate, old creams and/or loose dead tissue.
Gently but thoroughly clean the surface of the burn wounds.	To assist with wound cleansing.
If any blisters are present, using the sterile scissors, burst and deroof them expelling the fluid that has collected beneath.	Deroofing the blister removes any dead tissue that may harbour micro-organisms (Lawrence, 1989) and enables the nurse to assess the depth of the wound. Blister fluid retards healing by impairing local immunity (Rockwell and Ehrlich, 1990; Anon, 1990)
Using the forceps, lift up any loose or dead tissue and using the scissors cut off as close to the skin as possible.	
Assess the burn and treat according to the doctor's instructions:	
– Apply a layer of antibacterial cream, e.g. Silver Sulphadiazine onto the burn areas.	Silver Sulphadiazine cream is a topical antibacterial agent indicated as an adjunct for the prevention and treatment of wound sepsis in patients with partial and full thickness burns (Hoffman, 1984; Kemble and Lamb, 1987).

Action	Rationale
– Cover with the dressing of choice, either: Plastic bag (refer to appropriate procedure). Goretex bag (refer to appropriate procedure).	Plastic/Goretex bags are effective dressings for burns involving the hands and feet (Muddiman, 1989; Terill, Kedwards and Lawrence, 1991; Slater and Hughes, 1971; Kemble and Lamb, 1987).
2–3 layers of paraffin gauze and cover with layers of sterile gauze swabs.	Paraffin gauze is a vaseline impregnated gauze applied as a non-stick dressing (Thomas, 1994) and maintains a moist environment conducive to wound healing.
Secure the dressings in place with crepe bandage and adhesive tape.	To prevent the dressing from becoming displaced. Tape is preferable to pins for the safety of the patient.
Remove gloves and wash hands.	
Record in the appropriate documentation.	To maintain an accurate record.
Monitor and record the circulation to the extremities/limbs noting warmth, colour, pulses and sensation. Inform the doctor of any abnormalities.	To detect early signs of complications.
Assist the doctor with an escharotomy (see appropriate procedure) if required.	To accommodate the swelling and permit blood flow to the distal areas (Kemble and Lamb, 1987; Trofino and Orr, 1991).
Repeat the procedure and maintain wound assessments every 24–48 hours. (If skin grafting is required refer to the appropriate procedure.)	To promote healing, minimise the risk of infection and to monitor the evaluation of treatment. In the majority of cases, patients require surgical debridement of electrical burn wounds to remove dead tissue.

References

Anon (1990) Should burn blisters be burst? Emergency Medicine 22 (11): 57–9.

Arturson G, Hedlund A (1984) Primary treatment of 50 patients with high tension electrical injuries. Scandinavian Journal of Plastic Reconstructive Surgery 18: 111.

Baxter C (1970) Present concepts in the management of major electrical injury Surgical Clinics of North America 50: 1401.

Burke JF, Quinby WC, Bordoc C (1977) Patterns of high tension electrical injury in children and adolescents and their management. American Journal of Surgery 133: 492.

Butler ED, Grant TD (1977) Electrical injuries with special reference to the upper extremities. A review of 182 cases. American Journal of Surgery 134: 95.

Christiensen JA, Sherman RT, Bills GA et al. (1980) Delayed neuralgic injury secondary to high voltage current with recovery. Journal of Trauma 20: 166.

Fried M, Rosenburg B, Tuchman I, Ben-Hur N, Yardeni P, Sternberg N, Golan J (1991) Electrical burn injury of the scalp. Journal of the International Society for Burn Injuries 17 (4): 338–339.

Gordon MW, Reid WH, Awaad AM (1986) Electrical burns — incidence and prognosis in western Scotland. Burns Journal 12: 254.

Hanumadass ML, Voora SB, Kagan RJ et al. (1986) Acute electrical burns: A 10 year experience. Burns Journal 12: 427.

Hoffman S (1984) Silver sulphadiazine cream an antibacterial agent for topical use in burns. A review of the literature. Scandinavian Journal of Plastic and Reconstructive Surgery 18: 119.

Holliman CJ, Saffle JR, Kravitz M et al. (1982) Early surgical decompression in the management of electrical injuries. American Journal of Surgery 144: 733.

Kemble JVH, Lamb B (1987) Practical burns management. London: Hodder and Stoughton. pp 83–8.

Koller J (1991) High tension electrical arc-induced thermal burns caused by railway overhead cables. Burns Journal 17: 411.

Lawrence JC (1989) Management of burns. The Dressing Times 2 (3): 1–4.

Lee WR (1961) A clinical study of electrical accidents. British Journal of Industrial Medcine 18: 260.

Lee RC, Kolodney MS (1987a) Electrical injury mechanisms. Dynamics of the thermal response. Plastic and Reconstructive Surgery 80: 663.

Lee RC, Kolodney MS (1987b) Electrical injury mechanisms. Electrical breakdown of cell membranes. Journal of Plastic and Reconstructive Surgery 80: 672.

Muddiman R (1989) A new concept in hand burn dressings. Nursing Standard Special Supplement Sept, 23: 1–4.

Nichter LS, Bryant CA, Kerney JG et al. (1984) Injuries due to commercial electrical current. Journal of Burn Care and Rehabilitation 5: 124.

Reiche M, Kay S (1985) Electrical injuries due to railway high tension cables. Burns Journal 11: 423.

Rockwell C, Ehrlich D (1990) Should burn blisters be burst? Journal of Burn and Rehabilitation 11: 93.

Sances A, Larson SJ, Mykleburst J et al. (1979) Electrical injuries. Surgery, Gynaecology and Obstetrics 149: 97.

Shen ZY, Chang ZD, Wang NZ (1990) Electrical injury of the wrists: classification and treatment. A clinical analysis of 90 cases. Burn Journal 16: 449.

Slater RM, Hughes NC (1971) A simplified method of treating burns of the hands. British Journal of Plastic Surgery 24: 296.

Solem L, Fisher RP, Strate RG (1977) The natural history of electrical injury. Journal of Trauma 17: 487.

Sturim HS (1971) The treatment of electrical injuries. Journal of Trauma 11: 959.

Szabo K, Ver P (1983) Bone marrow aplasia after high voltage electrical injury. Burns Journal 10: 184.

Terrill PJ, Kedwards SM, Lawrence JC (1991) The use of Goretex bags for hand burns. Burns Journal 17 (2): 161–5.

Thomas S (1994) Jelonet. In Thomas S (Ed) Handbook of Wound Dressings. London: MacMillan. pp 98–9.

Trofino RB, Orr PM (1991) Types of burn. In Trofino RB, (Ed) Nursing Care of the Burn Injured Patient. Philadelphia: FA Davis Company. pp 34–6.

Wang XW, Roberts BB, Zapta-Stirvent RL (1985) Early vascular grafting to prevent upper extremity necrosis after electrical burns. Burns Journal 11: 359.

Wilson GR, Fowler CA, Housden PL (1987) A new burn area assessment chart. Burns Journal 13 (5): 401–5.

Wilson FR, French G (1987) Plasticised polyvinylchloride as a temporary dressing for burns. British Medical Journal 294: 256–7.

Zhu ZX, Yu DC, Wang Y, Zhoo L (1993) Successful treatment of a severe electrical injury involving the stomach. Journal of the International Society of Burn Injuries 19 (1): 80–2.

Further Reading

Bingham HG (1980) Electrical injuries to the upper extremity. Burns Journal 7: 155.

Housinger TA, Green L (1985) Myocardial damage in electrical injuries. Journal of Trauma 25: 122.

Lazarus HM, Hutton W (1982) Electric burns and frost bite. Journal of Trauma 22: 581.

Robson MC, Murphy RC, Heggers JP (1984) Progressive tissue loss in electrical injuries. Journal of Plastic and Reconstructive Surgery 73: 431.

Chapter 13
Care of patient with a chemical burn injury

Types of chemical burn injuries are usually related to geography, industry and the culture of the population (Trofino and Orr, 1991). Toxic chemical products used in military science, agriculture, industry and the home are all capable of producing a severe burn injury. The injuries involve tissue destruction by precipitation of chemical compounds in the cell, cellular dehydration, and the dissolution of tissue proteins (Trofino and Orr, 1991).

In general terms acid burns result in coagulation, necrosis and immediate pain whilst alkaline burns cause liquefaction necrosis with deeper penetration and less pain. The extent and depth of the burn injury is related to the concentration of the chemical, the activity and penetration of the substance, the duration of contact and the resistance of the tissues exposed.

Immediate treatment is to stop the burning process. Copious irrigation with water or saline is recommended and clothing should be removed as soon as possible. Nurses need to use protective clothing and rubber gloves. The patient's clothing should be placed in a heavy duty plastic bag and labelled. Any dry chemicals should be brushed off the surface of the skin prior to irrigation. Copious irrigation for 20–30 minutes decreases the rate of reaction between the tissues and the chemical. Neutralising agents are not recommended for initial use as precious time may be lost while the chemical continues to destroy tissues.

Chemical burns can be deceptive in their initial assessment and most are more serious than they appear to be. Tissue destruction may continue for up to 72 hours post injury.

1. Care of a patient with bitumen burns on admission to the Burns Unit

The circumstances surrounding hot tar burns are predictable. Many of these injuries are preventable and result from unsafe practices and/or equipment. Simple, basic preventative measures such as wearing protective clothing or carrying hot tar in containers with lids are recommended (Renz and Sherman, 1994).

Hot bitumen is used mainly to surface roads, for tiling roofs, waterproofing cars and in other industries (Juma, 1994). Many substances have been used to remove this sticky compound including butter (Schiller, 1983; Tiernan and Harris, 1993), mayonnaise (Shea and Fannon, 1981) and De-Solv-it: a citrus petroleum distillate with surfactant and lanolin (Stratta et al., 1983).

Bitumen is made from distillates of petroleum composed of long-chain hydrocarbons and waxes (Ashbell et al., 1967). When used for roof tiling or paving, the bitumen is heated to 140° C and when it splatters cools to 93° C (Ashbell et al., 1967; Stratta et al., 1983). On contact with the skin bitumen adheres, cools and solidifies (Renz and Sherman, 1994) and results in a deep burn due to heat transfer. It is sterile on impact and then acts as an occlusive dressing (Renz and Sherman, 1994). The skin beneath the bitumen then becomes colonised by organisms from the surrounding intact skin. The resulting high infection rate associated with these injuries has been reported in the literature (Ashbell et al., 1967; Stratta et al., 1983) and possibly promotes the conversion of partial thickness burns to full thickness burns (Stratta et al., 1983; Halfacre et al., 1981). In the first instance, initiate first aid treatment to reduce the effect of the thermal injury (Schiller, 1983; Stratta et al., 1983; Demling, Buerstatte and Perea, 1980) (Refer to appropriate procedure for advice.)

See sections 1–5 in Chapter 1 for advice on procedures.

Equipment

Trolley
Sterile dressing pack
1 pair of unsterile gloves
2 pairs of sterile gloves
Sachet of saline and alcohol swab
Gauze swabs
Sterile towel
Baby oil, mineral oil or liquid paraffin
Wound dressing (of choice)
Patient's prescription chart
Disposal bag

Action	Rationale
Administer analgesia as prescribed 30 minutes prior to commencing the procedure.	To minimise pain and discomfort for the patient.
Apply unsterile gloves.	For the protection of the nurse and to minimise the risk of cross infection.
Remove existing dressing and discard in the disposal bag.	To allow access to the wound site and to minimise the risk of cross infection.
Remove gloves and wash hands.	To minimise the risk of cross infection.

Action	Rationale
Treatment regimes may vary.	Removal of tar from the skin without inflicting further injury can be a challenging problem (Renz and Sherman, 1994).
– Leave the bitumen to solidify and then peel it off (Kemble and Lamb, 1987).	To facilitate removal of the bitumen. However, assessing the depth of the injury is difficult and the process may result in longer hospital stay with a consequent impact on hospital resources and the time taken by the patient to return to work (Juma, 1994). Also it does not allow proper skin cleansing and debridement and encourages bacterial proliferation (Renz and Sherman, 1994).
or – Instigate mechanical removal of the bitumen. or	To facilitate removal, however this can be both painful and traumatic (Juma, 1994).
– Apply sterile gloves and apply butter, baby oil, mineral oil or liquid paraffin directly onto the bitumen and massage gently into the skin.	Butter is non-toxic and is effective in removing bitumen with minimal discomfort to the patient (Tiernan and Harris, 1993). Baby oil/liquid paraffin is gentle and non toxic and dissolves the bitumen on contact, facilitating swift, painless removal of the bitumen and allowing early assessment of the depth of the burn (Juma, 1994).
Moisten the gauze swabs with saline and gently wipe over the skin.	To remove softened bitumen and allow access to the burn wound site.
Repeat the process every 4–8 hours until the bitumen has been removed from the skin.	To remove the bitumen and to allow access to the burn wound site (Renz and Sherman, 1994).
Remove gloves and wash hands.	
Apply sterile gloves and if the burn is on a limb place on a sterile towel.	To minimise the risk of cross infection.
Using the sterile scissors burst and deroof any blisters.	To maintain asepsis. Bursting and deroofing blisters allows removal of dead skin that may harbour micro-organisms (Lawrence, 1989).
Using the forceps lift up any loose dead tissue and using the sterile scissors cut as close to the skin as possible.	Dead tissue may provide a focus for micro-organisms.
If the wound appears red, inflamed or smells or is oozing purulent discharge take a bacteriological wound swab for culture and sensitivity, label and send to the microbiology laboratory.	To detect for early signs of infection.

Action	Rationale
Assess the wound and record on the appropriate documentation.	To determine the depth of the burn and percentage body surface area involved. (Wilson, Fowler and Housden, 1987).
Determine the type of wound dressing to be used.	To enhance wound healing.
Apply the wound dressing of choice adhering to the appropriate procedure.	To facilitate appropriate application and to maintain asepsis.
Document the wound dressing on the patient's prescription chart.	In accordance with unit policy/procedure for nurses prescribing wound care products.
Record in the patient's documentation.	To maintain an accurate record.

2. Care of a patient with cement burns on admission to the Burns Unit

Cement burns were first documented by Rowe and Williams (1963). Since then cement as a cause of burns has been well documented (Vickers and Edwards, 1976; Whiting, 1977; Fisher, 1979; Skundzulewski, 1980; Wilson and Davidson, 1985).

There are three factors in the aetiology of a cement burn — alkalinity, abrasion and duration of contact. All three of these factors are required to produce a burn (Wilson and Davidson, 1985). Plastic concrete has a pH of 12.4–12.7 and this alkalinity is created by the reaction of water and cement powder. Plastic concrete is a mixture of cement powder, coarse aggregate, sand and water in various proportions, thus concrete has an abrasive particulate content (Wilson and Davidson, 1985). Cement burns occur on areas of the body where there has been chafing by clothing impregnated with alkali and the fine aggregate part of the concrete. Duration of contact is important; the alkali remains in the skin despite cleansing and is often progressive. Therefore early recognition and treatment of these burn injuries is required.

See sections 1–5 in Chapter 1 for advice on procedures.

Equipment

    Trolley
    Sterile dressing pack
    2 pairs of unsterile gloves
    1 pair of sterile gloves
    Acetic acid (optional)
    Sterile towel
    Metal forceps
    Wound dressing (of choice)
    Patient's prescription chart
    Disposal bag

Action	Rationale
Administer analgesia as prescribed, approximately 30 minutes prior to commencing the procedure.	To minimise pain and discomfort for the patient.
Apply unsterile gloves.	For the protection of the nurse and to minimise the risk of cross infection.
Remove existing dressing and discard in the disposal bag.	To allow access to the wound site and minimise the risk of cross infection.
Remove gloves and wash hands.	To minimise the risk of cross infection.
Apply second pair of unsterile gloves.	For the protection of the nurse and to minimise the risk of cross infection.
Treatment regimes may vary:	
– Remove all soiled wet clothing. Irrigate the affected parts with copious amounts of water. or	To prevent further damage to the skin. Alkalis are soapy and require large volumes of water to remove them from the skin (Wilson and Davidson, 1985). Brief washing of the affected areas may not be sufficient to remove the alkali.
– Irrigate the affected areas with a phosphate buffer solution. or	To alter the pH level of the cement (Feldberg, Regan and Roberts, 1992).
– Soak the affected areas with 0.5–1% acetic acid solution as per prescription chart.	Acetic acid solution is an alternative first aid treatment after cement contact burns (Wilson and Davidson, 1985).
Observe the skin for signs of redness, broken areas, burning sensation, skin irritation.	To assess the severity of the burn (Wilson and Davidson, 1985).
Observe the distribution of the affected areas, e.g. knees, calves, ankles.	The site is dependent on the task being performed at the time and the type of footwear (Feldberg, Regan and Roberts, 1992).
Repeat the process of irrigation as directed by the medical staff.	If the cement is not dislodged, it continues to burn (Feldberg, Regan and Roberts, 1992). Irrigation will prevent progression of the burn.
Remove gloves and wash hands.	To minimise the risk of cross infection.
Apply sterile gloves and if the burn is on a limb place on a sterile towel.	To maintain asepsis.
Using sterile forceps and scissors lift up any loose dead skin and cut as close to the skin as possible.	Dead tissue may provide a focus for micro-organisms (Lawrence, 1989).
Assess the wound and record on the appropriate documentation.	To determine the depth of the burn and percentage body surface areas involved (Wilson, Fowler and Housden, 1987).

Action	Rationale
Determine the type of wound dressing to be used.	To enhance wound healing.
Apply the wound dressing of choice adhering to the appropriate procedure.	To facilitate appropriate application and maintain asepsis.
Remove gloves and wash hands.	To minimise the risk of cross infection.
Document the type of wound dressing on the patient's prescription chart.	In accordance with unit policy/procedure for nurses prescribing wound care products.
Discuss with the patient the possibility of wound excision and skin grafting.	Full thickness burn injuries will require surgical intervention to heal the wound (Feldberg, Regan and Roberts, 1992; Wilson and Davidson, 1985).
Record events in the appropriate nursing documentation.	To maintain an accurate record.

3. Care of a patient with hydrofluoric acid burns on admission to the Burns Unit

Hydrofluoric acid has unique properties that make it attractive for a variety of industrial and household uses. Exposure to dilute and concentrated solutions of hydrofluoric acid can lead to severe pain and tissue necrosis (Dowbak, Rose and Rohrich, 1994). The extent of injury is dependent on the surface area involved, the concentration of the acid solution (Bertolini, 1992), and the duration of exposure.

Topical exposure to concentrated hydrofluoric acid frequently has a fatal outcome even with the exposure of as little as 2.5% body surface area (Bertolini, 1992). Survival after major exposure is facilitated by aggressive emergency management including wound irrigation, sub-eschar injection of Calcium Gluconate, monitored supplementation of serum calcium and prompt wound excision (Sheridan et al., 1995). Clearly the best approach is through prevention.

See Sections 1–5 in Chapter I for advice on procedures.

Equipment

Trolley
Sterile dressing pack
2 pairs of unsterile gloves
1 pair of sterile gloves
Gauze swabs
Sterile towel
Metal forceps
Wound dressing of choice
Patient's prescription chart
Calcium Gluconate preparation (of choice)
Disposal bag

Action	Rationale
Administer analgesia as prescribed 30 minutes prior to commencing the procedure.	To minimise pain and discomfort for the patient.
Apply unsterile gloves.	For the protection of the nurse and to minimise the risk of cross infection.
Remove existing dressing and discard in the disposal bag.	To allow access to the wound site and to minimise the risk of cross infection.
Remove gloves and wash hands.	To minimise the risk of cross infection.
Irrigate the affected areas with water for 15–20 minutes.	Effective decontamination techniques will remove acid from the skin surface (Dowbak, Rose and Rohrich, 1994). Irrigation for longer than 20 minutes will delay topical treatment without significant benefit (Upfal and Doyle, 1990).
With fingertip exposure, trim the nails as short as possible.	To facilitate adequate decontamination.
Apply Calcium Gluconate gel 2.5–5% topically (as per prescription chart) and massage into the affected area as required.	Calcium Gluconate gel is used to form insoluble salts with fluoride ions and to prevent tissue penetration (Dowbak, Rose and Rohrich, 1994).
Reapply Calcium Gluconate gel and massage into the affected area until pain is entirely relieved.	To minimise pain and discomfort for the patient. Continued applications minimise the risk of reversion.
If pain persists for longer than 45 minutes a doctor may administer:	
– A subdermal injection. Current recommendations are 0.5 ml 10% Calcium Gluconate per square cm of affected tissue (Bertolini, 1992) or – Intra-arterial Calcium Gluconate.	If pain relief is incomplete subdermal injections of Calcium Gluconate have proved to be effective (Vance et al., 1986; Anderson and Anderson, 1988; Blunt, 1964). Intra-arterial administration of Calcium Gluconate allows larger amounts of elemental calcium to be delivered, reducing the need for painful digital injections (Bertolini, 1992). Injections are painful and may compromise the vasculature in oedematous tissue (Vance et al., 1986; Bertolini, 1992; Anderson and Anderson, 1988).

Action	Rationale
Monitor calcium and electrolyte levels and observe for clinical evidence of tetany.	To determine blood levels of calcium and electrolytes. Evidence of tetany, Chvostek's sign and/or Trousseau's sign indicate hypocalcaemia.
If any evidence of tetany inform the medical staff immediately.	To ensure appropriate immediate treatment.
Prepare the patient for surgery as directed by the medical staff and repeat the above processes as directed.	To ensure prompt wound excision and appropriate surgical wound management. To minimise pain and discomfort for the patient and ensure appropriate immediate treatment.
Record in the patient's documentation.	To maintain an accurate record.

4. Care of a patient with phenol burns on admission to the Burns Unit

Phenol is an aromatic hydrocarbon derived from coal tar, discovered in 1834 and initially used in crude form for the treatment of sewerage (Pardoe et al., 1976). This chemical substance may also be referred to as phenic acid, phenolum, phenyl hydrate, carbolic acid or hydroxybenzene.

In instances of intoxication the cytotoxical effects induce cardiovascular symptoms, e.g. tachycardia, hypotension and ventricular arrhythmias (Miller, 1942). Tachypnoea, pulmonary oedema, respiratory arrest and convulsive seizures can also occur (Botta, Straith and Goodwin, 1988; Kimbrough, 1973), and nausea, vomiting and diarrhoea have been noted (Angel and Rogers, 1972).

Phenol burns and intoxications are life-threatening injures (Horch, Spilker and Stark, 1994). They may appear to be harmless burns but it is imperative to re-emphasise the hazardous and life-threatening effects of exposure to this specific substance. The ingestion of as little as 1 g has been reported to cause death and approximately 50% of all reported cases have a fatal outcome (Lucas and Lane, 1895; Stitt-Thomson, 1896; Abrahams, 1990; Cronin and Brauer, 1949; Soares and Tift, 1982; Turtle and Dolan, 1992).

See Sections 1–5 in Chapter I for advice on procedures.

Equipment

Trolley
Sterile dressing pack
2 pairs of unsterile gloves
1 pair of sterile gloves
Sterile towel

Metal forceps
Scissors
Wound dressing (of choice)
Patient's prescription chart
Disposal bag

Action	Rationale
Administer analgesia as prescribed, approximately 30 minutes prior to commencing the procedure.	To minimise pain and discomfort for the patient.
Apply unsterile gloves.	For the protection of the nurse and to minimise the risk of cross infection.
Remove existing dressing and discard in the disposal bag.	To allow access to the wound site and minimise the risk of cross infection.
Remove gloves and wash hands.	To minimise the risk of cross infection.
Apply second pair of unsterile gloves.	For the protection of the nurse and to minimise the risk of cross infection.
Treatment regimes may vary. Besides the use of water, the application of soap, oil, glycerine, alcohol and bicarbonate have been suggested.	To promote decontamination, to reduce phenol contact and potential phenol absorption through the skin (Conning and Hayes, 1970).
Irrigate the affected areas with copious amounts of water or glycerine.	Small amounts of water dilute the chemical and expand the area involved (Horch, Spilker and Stark, 1994). Glycerine is four times as effective as water (Horch, Spilker, Stark, 1994) in neutralising the effects of phenol burns.
Examine the oral cavity for white, painless lesions.	To determine the possibility of ingestion of phenol and to confirm oral and/or oesophageal burns.
Observe the patient for nausea, vomiting, hypotension, arrhythmias, lethargy, seizures or coma.	To confirm phenol intoxication (Goodman and Gilman, 1975; Macek, 1983).
Obtain a specimen of urine and test for proteinuria and uraemia noting anuria or oliguria and colour.	To determine the extent of liver and renal injury. Dark urine may denote phenol excretion and may lead to renal damage, i.e. in the glomeruli and the tubules (Stajduhar-Caric, 1968).
Observe the skin for signs of denaturation, and necrosis followed by gangrene.	Skin damage may result after prolonged contact with phenol (Conning and Hayes, 1970; Cooper and Hayes, 1970).

Action	Rationale
Observe the colour of the skin for dull grey discoloration and progression to black eschar with absence of pain in the affected areas.	Phenol burns are known to cause partial thickness burns (Horch, Spilker and Stark, 1994), but the chemical may have some local anaesthetic properties that allow extensive damage to occur before any pain is recognised (Saydjari et al., 1986).
Observe the skin for signs of dermatitis and depigmentation.	Dermatitis and/or depigmentation may develop long after contact with the chemical compound has ceased (McGuire and Hendee, 1971; Saunders, Geddes and Elliot, 1988).
Repeat the process of irrigation as directed by the medical staff.	To promote decontamination and minimise the risk of phenol absorption through the skin (Conning and Hayes, 1970).
Remove gloves and wash hands.	To minimise the risk of cross infection.
Apply sterile gloves and if the burn is on a limb place on a sterile towel.	To maintain asepsis.
Using sterile forceps and scissors lift up any loose dead skin and cut as close to the skin as possible.	Dead tissue may provide a focus for micro-organisms (Lawrence, 1989).
Assess the wound and record on the appropriate documentation.	To determine the depth of the burn and percentage body surface area involved (Wilson, Fowler and Housder, 1987).
Determine the type of wound dressing to be used.	To enhance wound healing.
Apply the wound dressing of choice adhering to the appropriate procedure.	To facilitate appropriate application and maintain asepsis.
Remove gloves and wash hands.	To minimise the risk of cross infection.
Document the type of wound dressing on the patient's prescription chart.	In accordance with the unit policy/procedure for nurses prescribing wound care products.
Record events in the appropriate nursing documentation.	To maintain an accurate record.

5. Care of a patient with phosphorous burns on admission to the Burns Unit

White phosphorus is used mainly for military purposes, but it is also found in industrial and agricultural chemicals and in fireworks (Mendelson, 1971; Arena, 1979). It causes deep thermal injuries (Ben-Hur and Appelbaum, 1975).

White phosphorus is fat soluble, glows in yellow-green light, melts at 44.2° C and ignites spontaneously at 34° C upon drying and exposure to the air (Eldad and Simon, 1991). White phosphorus particles can burn the skin surface or penetrate into deeper tissues. Destruction of tissue will continue as long as it is exposed to oxygen. It may also cause multi-organ failure because of its toxic effects on erythrocytes, liver, kidneys and the heart (Eldad et al., 1995).

In the past, various methods of treatment have been suggested to neutralise the toxic effects of white phosphorus and to reduce morbidity and mortality (Cohen, 1974; Kaufman, Ulmann and Har-Shai, 1988).

The need for rapid removal or neutralisation of active phosphorus from the wound is imperative to increase the chances of survival from this type of chemical burn injury (Eldad and Simon, 1991)

See sections 1–5 in Chapter 1 for advice on procedures.

Equipment

Trolley
Sterile dressing pack
2 pairs of unsterile gloves
1 pair of sterile gloves
Gauze swabs
Sterile towel
Metal forceps
Scissors
Water, saline or Hartmann's solution
Neutralising agent (of choice)
Wound dressing (of choice)
Patient's prescription chart
Disposal bag

Action	Rationale
Administer analgesia as prescribed approximately 30 minutes prior to commencing the procedure.	To minimise the pain and discomfort for the patient.
Apply unsterile gloves.	For the protection of the nurse and to minimise the risk of cross infection.
Remove existing dressing and discard in the disposal bag.	To allow access to the wound site and minimise the risk of cross infection.
Remove gloves and wash hands. Apply second pair of unsterile gloves.	To minimise the risk of cross infection.
Treatment regimes may vary:	

Action	Rationale
– Irrigate the affected area with copious amounts of water or apply cold water packs.	Copious amounts of water (Curreri, Asch and Pruitt, 1970; Mendelson, 1971; Chu, 1982; Konjoyan, 1983) are recommended to remove particles from the wound site (Kaufman, Ulmann and Har-Shai, 1988). Water is required as elemental phosphorus burns spontaneously upon drying and exposure to the air. Burning phosphorus in contact with the skin causes a lesion that progresses until all the phosphorous is consumed or deprived of oxygen. Water irrigation of the wound site also reduces damage to the liver and kidneys (Eldad et al., 1995).
or	
– Irrigate the affected area with saline or Hartmann's solution.	To remove particles from the wound site (Weinberger Ben-Basset and Kaplan, 1978; Kaufman, Ulman and Har-Shai, 1988).
Move the patient to a darkened room or dim the lighting.	The glare of phosphorus particles is easier to detect in darkness (Eldad et al., 1995).
– Using the metal forceps remove any visible white phosphorus particles.	To assist with mechanical removal (Eldad et al., 1995).
or	
– Irrigate the affected area with copper sulphate solution 1–5% as per prescription chart and, using the metal forceps, remove the particles.	Copper sulphate stains the particles black and makes recognition and removal easier (Eldad et al., 1995). However it is a toxic agent (Summerin, Walder and Moncrief, 1967) and more than 50 mg is dangerous to adults (Blackwell, 1967).
or	
– Apply copper sulphate emulsion 3% to the affected area as per prescription chart.	The emulsion will overcome the toxicity of the copper sulphate solution (Ben-Hur and Appelbaum, 1975).
or	
– Irrigate the affected area with a sodium bicarbonate solution as per prescription chart.	To neutralise the effects of the phosphoric acids produced in the wound (Pruitt, 1970). However, there is no proof, this method alters prognosis (Curreri, Asch and Pruitt, 1970).
Repeat the above process as directed by the medical staff.	To remove particles from the wound site (Kaufman, Ulman and Har-Shai, 1988) and neutralise the toxic effects.
Remove gloves and wash hands.	To minimise the risk of cross infection.
Apply sterile gloves and if the burn is on a limb place on a sterile towel.	To maintain asepsis.

Action	Rationale
Using sterile forceps and scissors lift up any loose dead tissue and cut as close to the skin as possible.	Dead tissue may provide a focus for micro-organisms (Lawrence, 1989).
Take a bacteriological wound swab for culture and sensitivity, label and send to the microbiology laboratory.	To detect early signs of infection.
Assess the wound and record on the appropriate documentation.	To determine the depth of the burn and the percentage body surface area involved (Wilson, Fowler and Housden, 1987).
Determine the type of wound dressing to be used.	To enhance wound healing.
Apply the wound dressing, adhering to the appropriate procedure.	To facilitate appropriate application and asepsis.
Remove gloves and wash hands.	To minimise the risk of cross infection.
Document the type of wound dressing used on the patient's prescription chart.	In accordance with the unit policy/procedure for nurses prescribing wound care products.
Prepare the patient for surgery as directed by the medical staff	Deeply embedded particles cannot be removed by external irrigation and urgent surgical intervention may be required (Eldad et al., 1995).
Observe the patient for signs and symptoms of haemolytic anaemia, heart failure or electrolyte balance disturbances.	To detect possible damage of various body organs (Curreri, Asch and Pruitt, 1970; Mozingo et al., 1989), haemolytic anaemia (Summerin Walder and Moncrief, 1967), heart failure or electrolyte disturbances (Ben-Hur and Appelbaum, 1975; Eldad and Simon, 1991; Konjoyan, 1983).
Record in the appropriate patient documentation.	To maintain an accurate record.

6. Care of a patient with sulphuric acid burns on admission to the Burns Unit

Mineral acid burns are one of the commonest types of chemical burns and of these, sulphuric acid and nitric acid account for the majority of cases. These injuries occur as a result of either industrial accidents, laboratory mishaps or are an act of vengeance where deliberate disfigurement is the intention (Husain, Hasanain and Kumar, 1989).

The severity of burn injury depends on the pH of the solution and the duration of contact (Lewis, 1959). Irreversible damage will occur if the pH is less than 2.5 or more than 11.5. When the hydrogen ions are neutralised the damage ceases.

See sections 1–5 in Chapter 1 for advice on procedures.

Equipment

    Trolley
    Sterile dressing pack
    2 pairs of unsterile gloves
    Sterile towel
    Metal forceps
    Scissors
    Wound dressing (of choice)
    Patient's prescription chart
    Disposal bag

Action	Rationale
Administer analgesia as prescribed approximateley 30 minutes prior to commencing the procedure.	To minimise pain and discomfort of the patient.
Apply unsterile gloves.	For the protection of the nurse and to minimise the risk of cross infection.
Remove existing dressing and discard into the disposal bag.	To allow access to the wound site and to minimise the risk of cross infection.
Remove gloves and wash hands.	To minimise the risk of cross infection.
Apply second pair of unsterile gloves. Treatment regimes may vary:	For the protection of the nurse and to minimise the risk of cross infection.
Irrigate the affected areas with copious amounts of soap and water (for at least one hour).	One hour of irrigation is recommended to wash off the injurious agent as thoroughly as possible (Husain, Hasanain and Kumar, 1989).
	Soap will help neutralise the acid as it is alkaline (Husain, Hasanain and Kumar, 1989).
Examine the skin for evidence of a bronze discoloration or black eschar.	Sulphuric acid causes local damage on the skin by coagulation of proteins and later by vascular thrombosis (Hummel, 1982). Bronze discoloration may indicate a deep dermal burn and black eschar full thickness burns (Husain, Hasanain and Kumar, 1989).
Observe the patient for signs and symptoms of acidosis and inform medical staff immediately.	With acid burns the patient is at risk of metabolic acidosis because of the direct absorption of the acid into the circulation (Hummel, 1982).

Action	Rationale
Administer intravenous sodium bicarbonate solution as prescribed by the medical staff	Sodium bicarbonate solution is given to correct the acidosis (Davies, 1982; Peaston, 1968).
Obtain a specimen of urine and test for haemoglobinuria, myoglobin, pH, and note any colour changes.	There is potential for renal damage following acid burns (Shen, Ham and Fleming, 1943). Large amounts of haemoglobin and myoglobin in the urine, the physiological response of the kidney to conserve water and renal ischaemia may combine to produce acute tubular necrosis (Husain, Hasanain and Kumar, 1989).
Record urine output on a fluid balance chart.	To maintain an accurate record.
Repeat the process of irrigation as directed by the medical staff. Sodium bicarbonate may be applied to the affected areas after thorough irrigation has been completed.	To maximise complete removal of the acid solution. Sodium bicarbonate may be used to assist with neutralisation (Husain, Hasanain and Kumar, 1989).
Remove gloves and wash hands.	To minimise the risk of cross infection.
Apply sterile gloves and if the burn is on a limb place on a sterile towel.	To maintain asepsis.
Using sterile forceps and scissors lift up any loose dead skin and cut as close to the skin as possible.	Dead tissue may provide a focus for micro-organisms (Lawrence, 1989).
Assess the wound and record on the appropriate documentation.	To determine the depth of the burn and percentage body surface area involved (Wilson, Fowler and Housden, 1987).
Determine the type of wound dressing to be used.	To enhance wound healing.
Apply the wound dressing of choice adhering to the appropriate procedure.	To facilitate appropriate application and maintain asepsis.
Remove gloves and wash hands.	To minimise the risk of cross infection.
Document the type of dressing on the patient's prescription chart.	In accordance with the unit policy/procedure for nurses prescribing wound care products.
Record the events in the appropriate nursing documentation.	To maintain an accurate record.

References

Abrahams R (1990) A fatal case of carbolic acid poisoning in an infant due to absorption by the skin. Paediatrics 9: 241.

Anderson WJ, Anderson JR (1988) Hydrofluoric acid burns on the hand. Mechanisms of injury and treatment. Journal of Hand Surgery 13A: 52–7.

Angel A, Rogers KJ (1972) An analysis of the consultant activity by substituted benzenes in the mouse. Toxicology Applied Pharmacology 21: 214.

Arena JM (1979) Poisoning Toxicology, Symptoms Treatment (4th edition) Springfield Il: Charles C Thomas. p 740.

Ashbell TS, Crawford HH, Adamson JE et al., (1967) Tar and grease removal from injured parts. Plastic Reconstructive Surgery 40: 330–1.

Ben-Hur N, Appelbaum J (1975) The phosphorus burn and its specific treatment. Burns Journal 1: 222-82.

Bertolini JC (1992) Hydrofluoric acid: a review of toxicity. Journal of Emergency Medicine 10: 163–8.

Blackwell OR (1967) Recommendations for safer treatment of white phosphorus burns. Tapei, Taiwan, Technical Report, Naval Medical Research 20 Sept.

Blunt CP (1964) Treatment of hydrofluoric acid burns by injection with calcium gluconate. Industrial Medicine 869–71.

Botta SA, Straith RE, Goodwin HH (1988) Cardiac arrhythmias in phenol face peeling — A suggested protocol for prevention. Aesthetic Plastic Surgery 12: 115.

Chu CS (1982) Burns update in China: II Special burn injury and burns of special areas. Journal of Trauma 22: 574.

Cohen SR (1974) A review of the health hazards from copper exposures. Journal of Occupational Medicine 16: 621–4.

Conning DM, Hayes MJ (1970) The dermal toxicity of phenol — An investigation of the most effective first aid measures. British Journal of Industrial Medicine 27: 155.

Cronin TD, Brauer RO (1949) Death due to phenol contained in foil. Journal of American Medical Association 139: 777.

Curreri PW, Asch MJ, Pruitt BA (1970) The treatment of chemical burns. Journal of Trauma 10: 634.

Davies JWL (1982) Physiological Response to Burn Injury. London: Academic Press. pp 230–5.

Demling RH, Buerstatte RPH, Perea A (1980) Management of hot tar burns. Journal of Trauma 20: 242.

Dowbak G, Rose K, Rohrich RJ (1994) A biochemical and histologic rationale for the treatment of hydrofluoric acid burns with calcium gluconate. Journal of Burn Care and Rehabilitation 15 (4): 323–7.

Eldad A, Simon GA (1991) The phosphorous burn — A preliminary comparative experimental study of various forms of treatment. Journal of the International Society for Burn Injuries 17: 198–200.

Eldad A, Wisoki M, Cohen H, Breiterman S, Chaouat M, Wexler MR, Ben-Bassat H (1995) Phosphorous burns evaluation of various modalities for primary treatment. Journal of Burn Care and Rehabilitation 16 (1): 49–55.

Feldberg L, Regan PJ, Roberts AHNR (1992) Cement burns and their treatment. Burns Journal 18 (1): 51–3.

Fisher AA (1979) Cement burns resulting in necrotic ulcers due to kneeling in wet cement. Cutis 23: 272–370.

Goodman L, Gilman AJ (1975) The Pharmacological Basis of Therapeutics (5th Edition) New York: MacMillan. p 990.

Halfacre S, Apesos J, Rodeheaver GT, Edlich RF (1981) Hot tar skin burns. Current Concepts in Trauma Care 18–9.

Horch R, Spilker G, Stark GB (1994) Phenol burns and intoxication. Journal of the International Society for Burn Injuries 20 (1): 45–50.

Hummel R (1982) Clinical Burns Therapy. New York: John Wright. pp 216–21.

Husain MT, Hasanain J, Kumar P (1989) Sulphuric acid burns — A report of a mass domestic incident. Burns Journal 15 (6): 389–91.

Juma A (1994) Bitumen burns and the use of baby oil. Burns Journal 20 (4): 363–635.

Kaufman T, Ulmann Y, Har-Shai Y (1988) Phosphorous burns: a practical approach to local treatment. Journal of Burn Care and Rehabilitation 9: 174–5.

Kemble JVH, Lamb BE (1987) Practical Burns Management. (1st Edition) London: Hodder and Stoughton.

Kimbrough RD (1973) Review of recent evidence of toxic effects of hexachlorophene. Paediatrics 51: 391.

Konjoyan TR (1983) White phosphorous burns, case report and literature review. Military Medicine 148: 881.

Lawrence JC (1989) Management of burns. The Dressing Times 2 (3): 1–4.

Lewis GK (1959) Chemical burns. American Journal of Surgery 98: 928.

Lucas RC, Lane WA (1895) Two cases of carbolic acid coma induced by application of carbolic acid compresses to the skin. Lancet i: 1362.

Macek C (1983) Venous thrombosis results from phenol injections. Journal American Medical Association 249: 1807.

McGuire J, Hendee J (1971) Biochemical basis for depigmentation of skin by phenolic germicides. Journal of Investigative Dermatology 57: 256.

Mendelson JA (1971) Some principles of protection against burns from flame and incendiary munitions. Journal of Trauma 11: 286

Miller FG (1942) Poisoning by phenol. Canadian Medical Association 46: 615.

Mozingo DW, Smith AA, McManus WF et al., (1989) Chemical burns. Journal of Trauma 10: 634–42.

Pardoe R, Minami RT, Sato RM, Schlesinger SL (1976) Phenol burns. Burns Journal 3: 29.

Peaston R (1968) Metabolic acidosis in burns. British Medical Journal 1: 809.

Pruitt BA (1970) Management of burns in the multiple injury patient. Surgical Clinics of North America 50: 1283.

Renz BM, Sherman R (1994) Hot tar burns, twenty seven hospitalised cases. Journal of Burn Care and Rehabilitation 15 (4): 341–5.

Rowe RJ, Williams GH (1963) Severe reaction to cement. Archives of Environmental Health 7: 709.

Saunders A, Geddes L, Elliot P (1988) Are phenolic disinfectants toxic to staff members? Australian Nurses Journal 17: 25.

Saydjari R, Abston S, Desai MH et al., (1986) Chemical Burns. Journal of Burn Care and Rehabilitation 7: 404.

Schiller WR (1983) Tar burns in the south west. Surgery, Gynaecology, Obstetrics. 157: 38.

Shea PC, Fannon P (1981) Mayonnaise and hot tar burns. Journal of the Medical Association 70: 659–60.

Shen SC, Ham TH, Flemming EM (1943) Studies on destruction of red blood cells. Mechanism and complications of haemoglobinaemia in patients with thermal burns. New England Journal of Medicine 229: 701.

Sheridan RL, Ryan CM, Quinby WC, Blair J, Tompkins RG, Burke JF (1995) Emergency management of major hydrofluoric acid exposures. Burns Journal 21 (1): 62–4.

Skundzulewski JJ (1980) Cement burns. Annals of Emergency Medicine 9: 316.

Soares ER, Tift JP (1982) Phenol poisoning — Three fatal cases. Journal of Forensic Science 27: 729.

Stajduhar-Caric Z (1968) Acute phenol poisoning. Journal of Forensic Medicine 15: 141.

Stitt Thomson J (1896) A case of fatal poisoning by carbolic acid. British Medical Journal 2: 194.

Stratta RJ, Saffle JR, Kravitz M et al. (1983) Management of tar and asphalt injuries. American Journal of Surgery 146: 766–9.

Summerin WT, Walder AL, Moncrief JA (1967) White phosphorous burns and massive haemolysis. Journal of Trauma 7: 476–84.

Tiernan E, Harris A (1993) Butter in the initial treatment of hot tar burns. Journal of the International Society for Burn Injuries 19 (5): 437–8.

Trofino RB, Orr PM (1991) Types of burns. In Trofino RB, (Ed) Nursing Care of the Burn Injured Patient. Philadelphia: FA Davis. pp 31–5.

Turtle WRM, Dolan T (1992) A case of rapid and fatal absorption of carbolic acid through the skin. Lancet ii: 1273.

Upfal M, Doyle C (1990) Medical management of hydrofluoric acid exposure. Journal of Occupational Medicine 32: 726–31.

Vance MV, Curry SC, Kunkel DB et al., (1986) Digital hydrofluoric acid burns. Treatment with intra-arterial calcium infusion. Annals of Emergency Medicine 15: 59–65.

Vickers HR, Edwards DH (1976) Cement burns. Contact Dermatitis 2: 73.

Weinberger A, Ben-Basset M, Kaplan I (1978) Treatment of phosphorous burns. Harefuah 94: 412.

Whiting RK (1977) Alkali burns caused by contact with cement. Palliative Medicine 80: 48.

Wilson GR, Davidson PM (1985) Full thickness burns from ready mixed cement. Burns Journal 12: 139–44.

Wilson GR, Fowler CA, Housden PL (1987) A new burn area assessment chart. Burns Journal 13 (5): 401–5.

Chapter 14
Monitoring vital signs of burn trauma patients

Caring for critically ill patients following burn trauma requires consistent observation and monitoring of vital signs. Recordings are generally made hourly; however, changes in the patient's condition may justify either more frequent recordings (e.g. during a period of instability) or less frequent recordings (e.g. during a period of stable recovery).

More frequent observations are required when burns patients undergo both invasive and non-invasive procedures. Vital signs must be monitored before, during and after procedures to ensure that changes in the patient's condition are immediately detected.

1. Procedure for fluid balance monitoring

Action	Rationale
Record and assess hourly:	
Oral fluids (especially in the case of children if a fluid restriction is in progress).	To minimise the risk of burn encephalopathy developing. (Antoon, Volpe, Crawford 1972). To ensure that the desired fluid balance is maintained.
Prescribed intravenous infusions and patency of lines.	To ensure desired fluid balance is maintained.
Infusion rates and volume of fluid delivered. Urine output:	To ensure the prescribed rate is administered at all times.
– Amount.	A urine output of 0.5–1 ml/kg body weight per hour must be achieved to reduce the risk of myoglobinuria and acute tubular necrosis (Wilmore et al., 1974).
– Colour.	Colour changes of the urine may indicate the presence of haemoglobinuria or myoglobinuria (Settle, 1986).
– Abnormalities such as blood, glucose and protein and note the specific gravity.	To determine the level of renal function and adequacy of fluid replacement.
– Calculate fluid balance.	To observe for fluid overload or inadequacy of fluid requirements.

Action	Rationale
Record and assess 4-hourly:	
Intravenous access site for signs of extravasation or infection.	Extravasation can lead to tissue necrosis. Infection may indicate the need to remove any intravenous device, e.g. a cannula.
Security of the intravenous lines.	Intravenous access may be difficult in patients with major burns, therefore line maintenance is vital.
Haematocrit measurements.	Haematocrit measurements are used to measure plasma deficit and indicate whether the patient is under or over hydrated (Settle, 1986).
Nasogastric aspirate.	To assess absorption of nasogastric (bolus) feeds and to assess gastric emptying (McDonald et al., 1991).
Drainage from any wound sites.	To determine the type and amount of fluid lost from additional sites.

2. Procedure for respiratory monitoring

Action	Rationale
Observe, record and assess: Respiratory rate (in accordance with the patient's age).	To detect any changes in the patient's respiratory condition. Abnormalities may indicate an inhalation injury or the need to reassess the use of respiratory depressing analgesia.
Air entry.	To detect any changes in the patient's respiratory condition.
Breath sounds — evidence of stridor, hoarseness, wheezing, dyspnoea, or cough.	Evidence may indicate clinical symptoms associated with an inhalation injury (Coiffi and Rue, 1991).
Colour of lips, skin and nail beds.	May indicate cyanosis (Torrance, 1992).
Oxygen saturation via pulse oximetry.	To detect early signs of hypoxia (Miller, 1992).
Arterial blood gases.	To assess respiratory function and gaseous exchange. These may be normal in the initial phase of management but will serve as a baseline (Coiffi and Rue, 1991).
Inspired oxygen level and percentage of oxygen prescribed.	To ensure the desired oxygen level is maintained.
Chest expansion.	Full thickness burns to the chest may restrict movement of the chest wall and lung expansion and the patient may need escharotomies to assist with breathing.

3. Procedure for temperature monitoring

Action	Rationale
Record and assess:	
Peripheral temperature either axillary, toe or groin.	To detect any changes in the patient's temperature. With a fall in peripheral temperature there will be peripheral vasoconstriction at the extremities and a drive towards heat conservation.
Core temperature.	To detect any changes in the patient temperature. To detect early signs of complications of Toxic Shock Syndrome (Frame et al. 1985).
– Rectal	This source maintains a close correlation with the core body temperature and is least affected by external variables (Fulbrook, 1993).
– Via temperature sensor (e.g. Foley catheter)	This method is less embarrassing for the patient and minimises discomfort.
– Via tympanic temperature sensor.	The tympanic area has an abundant arterial blood supply sensitive to core temperature changes (Closs, 1992). It is not recommended for use with patients who have sustained burns to the ears as they may find the sensor painful and uncomfortable.

4. Procedure for cardiovascular monitoring

Action	Rationale
Observe record and assess:	
Heart rate and rhythm.	To detect any changes in the patient's cardiovascular condition.
– Blood pressure — manually or via arterial line (if present).	To detect the patient's cardiovascular condition (Wilkie, 1992).
– ECG	To help to identify dysrhythmias and to assess the effects of fluid shift on cardiac status. To obtain baseline data (Foulkes, 1991).
– Cardiac rhythm	Assists in identifying and treating arrhythmias.

5. Procedure for the care of a child with a pyrexia of 39°C plus

A core pyrexia of 39°C in a child requires immediate treatment to prevent febrile convulsions. It may also be one of the first signs of burns encephalopathy (Antoon, Volpe and Crawford, 1972), if the skin temperature has not risen in conjunction with the core temprature. It is essential to find any possible cause for a hyperpyrexia and a full microbiological screen should be carried out to identify the cause.

See Sections 1 – 2 in Chapter 1 for advice on procedures.

Equipment

Rectal probe and temperature box
Thermometer
Bacteriological wound swabs
Urine bag (if not catheterised)
Universal container
Stool sample pot
Socially clean tray
Patient's prescription chart

Action	Rationale
Commence hourly monitoring of skin and rectal temperatures.	To monitor the child's temperature and note any deviation between skin and rectal temperatures.
Do not use fan or tepid sponge the child.	This will result in reducing the peripheral temperature only. When this happens the body tries to compensate by raising the core temperature.
If the rectal temprature rises administer suitable antipyretics as per prescription chart.	Antipyretics are effective in reducing the body temperature.
Inform the on call medical staff.	The medical staff may wish to take blood cultures.
Commence a full bacteriological screen to include wound, ear, nose and throat swabs and stool and urine specimens. Label and send to the microbiology laboratory for culture and sensitivity.	To identify any infection that may be causing the pyrexia (Frame et al. 1985).
Observe and record other signs of infection, e.g. pain, redness, swelling, diarrhoea, presence of pus, foul smelling urine, sore throat, earache.	In order to help to identify source of infection.

Action	Rationale
Regulate the room temperature and amount of blankets in accordance with the skin temperature.	This will either cool or warm the skin as appropriate.
Aim to keep the skin and rectal temperatures within at least 2°C of each other.	Any divergence may indicate burns encephalopathy. Once the temperatures begin to diverge it is difficult to bring them together again.
Record in the appropriate documentation.	To maintain an accurate record.

References

Antoon AY, Volpe JJ, Crawford JD (1972) Burn encephalopathy in children. Paediatrics 50 (4): 609–16.

Closs J (1992) Monitoring the body temperature of surgical patients. Surgical Nurse 5 (1): 12–16.

Coiffi WG, Rue LW (1991) Diagnosis and treatment of inhalation injuries. Critical Care. Nursing Clinics of North America. 3 (2): 191–8.

Foulkes J (1991) ECG. What, how, why? Surgical Nurse 4 (4): 14–19.

Frame JD, Eve MD, Hackett MEJ, Dowsett EG, Brainan-Gault DT, Wilmhurst AD (1985) The toxic shock syndrome in burned children. Burns Journal. 11: 234–41.

Fulbrook P (1993) Core temperature measurements in adults — A literature review. Journal of Advanced Nursing 18: 1451–60.

McDonald US, Claibourne W, Sharp JR, Deitch EA (1991) Immediate enteral feeding in burn patients is safe and effective. Annals of Surgery. February issue: 177–83.

Miller P (1992) Using pulse oximetry to take clinical nursing decisions. Orthopaedic Nursing 4: 39–42.

Settle JAD (1986) Burns. The First Five Days. Essex UK: Smith and Nephew, Pharmaceuticals.

Torrance C (1992) Respiratory observations. Surgical Nurse 5 (3): 22–5.

Wilkie AV (1992) Blood pressure monitoring. Surgical Nurse 5 (2): 18–22.

Wilmore DW et al. (1974) Alterations in hypothalmic function following thermal injury. Journal of Trauma 15: 697.

Further Reading

Childs C (1994) Temperature regulation in burned patients. British Journal of Intensive Care. April Issue 129–34.

Emery JL, Campbell-Reid DA (1962) Cerebral oedema and spastic hemiplegia following minor burns in young children. British Journal of Surgery 50: (219) 53–6.

Kay S, Samba-Siva RG, Lord D, Greenhough S (1986) Intracranial pressure monitoring as an aid to resuscitation in the burnt and asphyxiated child. Burns Journal 12: 212-13.

McManus WF, Hunt JL, Pruitt BA (1974) Post burn consultative disorder in children. Journal of Trauma 14: 396–401.

Rainbow C (1989) Monitoring the Critically Ill Patient. London: Heinemann Nursing. pp 78-101.

Warlow CP, Hinton P (1969) Early neurological disturbances following relatively minor burns in young children. Lancet 2: 978–82.

Chapter 15
The use of haematocrit measurements in patients following burn trauma

Immediately after a burn injury occurs the capillaries become more permeable — water, electrolytes and albumin leak out of the circulation onto the surface of the burn as exudate, into the extravascular space as oedema, and into the dermis as blisters.

The result is a reduced volume of plasma in the circulation and this may be referred to as hypovolaemic shock. At the same time this occurs the red blood cells in the circulation become concentrated, the blood increases in viscosity and the circulation slows down.

The body will initially compensate by reducing the blood supply to the skin, gut and kidneys but if this situation continues untreated the results of shock may be fatal.

The severity of the shock is related not to the cause or depth of the burn but to the body surface area involved in the burn injury. Children with over 10% body surface area (BSA) burns and adults with over 15% (BSA) burns rapidly develop hypovolaemic shock. Therefore, intravenous fluid resuscitation of plasma is a priority in treatment to increase the circulating volume and to restore and maintain adequate perfusion to all tissues of the body.

The volume of fluid to be given is calculated using the Muir and Barclay (1962) formula:

$$\frac{\text{Weight of patient (kgs)} \quad \times \quad \% \text{ BSA burns}}{2} \quad = \quad \text{Volume of plasma per period (ml)}$$

The first 36 hours is divided into periods of 4, 4, 4, 6, 12 hours and the calculated volume of plasma is infused in each period.

Initially, intravenous fluids are administered at a fast rate to correct the existing plasma deficits but this is gradually reduced over the 36 hour resuscitation period. The formula should only be used as a guide and the patient should be carefully monitored and fluids altered according to the patient's condition (Muir, Barclay and Settle, 1987). One method of monitoring whether adequate volumes of plasma are being administered is to measure the haematocrit packed cell volume (Kemble and Lamb,

1987). On admission to the Burns Unit a capillary blood sample is obtained from the patient, centrifuged and the ratio of red blood cells to plasma is measured on a scale. Normal values are as follows (Settle, 1986):

6 months	=	36%
1 – 3 years	=	38%
4 – 5 years	=	39%
6 – 10 years	=	40%
11 – adult (females)	=	40%
11 – adult (males)	=	41–44%

If plasma has been lost (and not adequately replaced) there is a higher proportion of red blood cells and the haematocrit count will be high, therefore more fluid will be required (Morgan, 1991).

If a higher proportion of plasma to red cells is observed the haematocrit count will be low, therefore less fluid is required (Vaccaro and Trofino, 1991).

This procedure will be repeated 4 hours after the initial injury occurred, then at the end of two further 4-hour periods, two 6-hour periods and one 12-hour period (to complete the 36 hour resuscitation period following a burn injury). If, during any one of these periods, monitoring the haematocrit shows too much or too little fluid is being given the fluid volumes are adjusted accordingly.

N.B. An alternative method of monitoring the state of the circulation at any time is to calculate the actual volume of plasma missing from the circulation. Use the haematocrit measurement and apply the following formula (Settle, 1986):

$$\text{Deficit} = \text{Blood volume} \left[\text{blood volume} \times \frac{\text{normal haematocrit}]}{\text{observed haematocrit}]} \right.$$

1. Procedure for obtaining a blood sample for haematocrit measurement

See sections 1, 2 and 5 in Chapter 1 for advice on procedures and sharps policy.

Equipment

Small clean tray
1 pair of unsterile gloves
Minilet (lancet)
Gauze swab
Capillary tubes
Crystoseal
Centrifuge machine
Haematocrit measure
Ruler (optional)
Sharps box

Action	Rationale
Place minilet, gauze swab, capillary tubes and crystoseal onto a tray.	To prepare correct equipment for the patient's bedside.
Take the tray to the patient and explain procedure.	Information can reduce anxiety and help a person cope with a stressful situation (Lazarus and Averill, 1972).
Ensure the area where blood is to be taken from is clean, warm and not the site of a burn.	To minimise the risk of infection and ensure a good blood supply.
A sample of blood can be obtained from the fingertip, toe or earlobe.	These areas usually have a good blood supply.
Apply unsterile gloves.	To protect the nurse from blood-borne infections.
Hold the area firmly between thumb and index finger to create a degree of engorgement.	To encourage a good blood supply to the area before puncturing the skin.
Using the minilet, puncture the area with a brisk firm action.	To puncture the skin sufficiently to obtain enough blood to fill the capillary tube.
With gentle pressure squeeze a large drop of blood onto the surface of the skin.	To allow the capillary tube to be filled from one large drop of blood and to minimise air collecting and blood clotting in the capillary tube before it is full.
Place the open end of the capillary tube into the blood, hold downwards and repeat as above until the tube is full (if there is enough blood fill two tubes).	Gravity aids the filling of the capillary tube. Filling two tubes is a safety measure in case one is damaged in the centrifuge machine.
Seal the unfilled end of the capillary tube by pushing the end at a 90° angle into the crystoseal. Twist and remove the sealed tube.	To prevent blood spilling out of the capillary tube when it is being centrifuged.
Cover the skin puncture area with a gauze swab and apply gentle pressure until the area stops bleeding.	To stop bleeding and to prevent haematoma formation.
Dispose of minilet needle into the sharps box.	To minimise the risk of needle stick injuries.
Take the filled and sealed capillary tube(s) to the centrifuge machine.	To allow the blood to be processed.

2. Procedure for using the centrifuge machine

Action	Rationale
Raise the outer lid of the centrifuge machine.	To allow access.
Unscrew inner lid and lift off.	To allow access to lower spinning section.
Place two capillary tubes in the centrifuge machine opposite each other.	To balance the centrifuge machine.
Replace inner lid and screw on tightly.	To prevent the capillary tubes moving while the centrifuge is operating.
Lower the outer lid.	To cover the spinning section. The centrifuge machine will not start unless securely closed.
Set the timer to 5 minutes.	Time required to ensure plasma and cells are separated.
Wait for the centrifuge to stop spinning before lifting the outer lid.	If the lid is raised when the centrifuge machine is spinning there is a risk of injuring fingertips.
Unscrew inner lid and lift off.	To allow access to the capillary tubes.
Remove the capillary tubes from the centrifuge machine.	To prepare for reading the result.
Clean the centrifuge with hot water and detergent (if required), replace lids.	To minimise the risk of cross infection from spillage of blood. To prepare the centrifuge for further use.

3. Procedure for reading the haematocrit sample result

Equipment

Capillary tube(s)
Haematocrit measure
Ruler (optional)

Action	Rationale
Place the haematocrit measure on a flat surface in good light.	To enable an accurate result to be obtained.
Place the capillary tube into the groove of the plastic slider on the haematocrit measure.	To ensure the capillary tube is secured into position and to facilitate an accurate reading.
– Place the bottom of the red blood cell level on the black line at the base. Place the top of the plasma level on the top black line.	

Action	Rationale
– Move the plastic slide along until the top and bottom lines coincide with the appropriate marks on the measure.	
– Slide the black knob on the left side up until the silver line is at the divide between the plasma and the red blood cells.	To identify the separating line between the plasma and red blood cells.
– Note the number corresponding to the silver line on the right hand side and record the reading.	The number denotes the haematocrit reading and is recorded as a percentage.
– If there is insufficient blood to use the haematocrit measure, use the millimetre scale on a ruler.	To obtain the haematocrit result without taking further blood from the patient.
– Measure the number of red blood cells in millimetres, divide by the total length of the sample and multiply by 100.	To estimate the haematocrit result.

Red cells	plasma	
12 mm		$12/43 \times 100 = 28\%$

43 mm

Dispose of the capillary tube into the sharps box.	In accordance with unit sharps policy
Repeat the procedure if the result obtained seems inappropriate for the age of the patient and/or has significantly changed from the previous result(s).	To maintain an accurate result (for normal values refer to introductory section).
Record the result in the appropriate documentation.	To maintain an accurate record.

References

Kemble JVH, Lamb BE (1984) Plastic Surgical and Burns Nursing. 1st Edition. Eastbourne: Baillière Tindall. pp 34, 64.

Kemble JVH, Lamb BE (1987) Practical Burns Management. London: Hodder and Stoughton p 238.

Morgan B (1991) Pathology of burns. In: Leverage A, (Ed) Therapy for the Burn Patient London: Chapman and Hall. p 14.

Muir IFK, Barclay TL (1962) Treatment of burns shock. In Muir IFK, Barclay TL (Eds) Burns and Their Treatment. London: Lloyd-Luke. pp 14–54.

Muir IFK, Barclay TL, Settle JAD (1987) Burns and their treatment. (3rd Edition). London: Butterworth.

Settle JAD (1986) Burns — The First Five Days, Essex, UK: Smith and Nephew Pharmaceuticals. pp 13–15.

Vaccaro P, Trofino RB (1991) Care of the patient with minor to moderate burns. In Trofino RB, (Ed) Nursing Care of the Burn Injured Patient. Philadelphia: FA Davis. p 120.

Further Reading

Kemble JVH, Lamb BE (1984) Plastic Surgical and Burns Nursing. 1st Edition. Eastbourne: Baillière Tindall. p 379.

Lazarus RS, Averill JR (1972) Emotion and condition academic. In Spielberger CD. (Ed) Anxiety: Current Trends in Theory and Research. New York: Academic Press.

Chapter 16
Care of a patient requiring an intravenous infusion

Intravenous cannulation is used for replacing fluids, crystalloids, blood and blood products. Following burn trauma the use of intravenous therapy is advised for all children with over 10% body surface area burns and all adults with over 15% body surface area burns.

During the first 36 hours of fluid resuscitation the fluid of choice is human plasma protein fraction solution. The aim of infusion therapy is first to replace any current deficit of plasma loss and second to match the loss hour by hour until the plasma leak ceases, thereby minimising the risk of hypovolaemic shock.

The formula used to predict the likely fluid requirement and indicate an appropriate rate of infusion was devised by Muir and Barclay (1962):

$$\frac{\text{Weight of patient (kg)} \times \text{\% BSA burns}}{2} = \text{Volume of plasma per period (ml)}$$

(The first 36 hours after a burn injury are divided into six successive periods, 4, 4, 4, 6, 6, and 12 hours. The formula is used to calculate equal volumes of plasma per period (Settle, 1986).)

A second infusion may also be commenced to replace metabolic water requirements and this is usually 4% dextrose with 0.18% saline, the volume calculated according to the patient's weight.

As Finch (1982) says: "It is important to remember that all cannulation procedures put the vascular compartment into direct communication with the external environment and partly neutralise the protective effect of an intact epithelial surface." And Jenner (1983) wrote: "Intravenous infusion therapy is a common but potentially dangerous procedure and it is important that we should be aware of the sources of infection so that we can minimise the risks."

Asepsis, safety and comfort, are important principles that should be applied to all aspects of intravenous care.

Selection of a vein and insertion of the cannula

This is carried out by a doctor or a nurse trained in the procedure who will select the site, insert the cannula and commence the infusion. The non-dominant upper limb is usually the site of choice, unless both arms are severely burned when it is recommended that a large vein in either forearm or anticubital fossa should be used. (In some cases intravenous cut down may be required). In either case the largest possible cannula should be inserted (to allow for an adequate flow rate) and secured safely in position to minimise the risk of dislodging and losing intravenous access which may affect the patient's life.

Use of an air inlet

Some rigid containers require the use of an air inlet. In these circumstances it is best to select a giving set which incorporates an air inlet. If a separate air inlet is used, care must be taken to ensure the filter does not become wet, as this allows airborne micro-organisms to enter the system and constitutes a 'break' in a closed system. If this occurs the infusion fluid and the administration set must be discarded and replaced. A hypodermic needle must not be used (Allwood, 1981).

1. Procedure for setting up an intravenous infusion

See sections 1–5 in Chapter 1 for advice on procedures and sharpes policy.

Equipment

Trolley
Sterile dressing pack
Povidone Iodine solution 10% with alcohol or Chlorhexidine 0.5% (red) with
    alcohol
Cannula — various sizes
Semi-permeable film dressing
Hypo-allergenic tape
Patient's prescription chart
Prescribed intravenous fluid
Intravenous administration set
Dripstand or infusion controller
Tourniquet (size appropriate to patient)
5 ml syringe/needle
5 ml ampoule normal saline
Specimen bottles (if blood samples required)
Label for 'administration set' change
Fluid balance chart
Clean scissors (if required)
Sharps box

Action	Rationale
Examine the selected limb, clip away hair if necessary, while holding the scissors parallel to the skin.	To allow the dressing to stick. Clipping the hair is preferable to shaving which is likely to cause microscopic abrasions so creating a potential entry site for micro-organisms (Hamilton, Hamilton and Lane, 1977).
Open the sterile dressing pack and using the 5 ml syringe and needle draw up 5 ml normal saline.	To maintain asepsis and to prepare the saline flush for use.
Clean the skin with the appropriate agent and allow to air dry.	To minimise the risk of infection (Lamb, 1993).
Insert the cannula and check patency using the saline flush.	To ensure the correct positioning of the cannula.
Secure the cannula with the semi-permeable film dressing.	To protect the wound from contamination and to allow easy viewing of the cannula site (Keenlyside, 1992).
Examine the fluid, outer wrapper and inner container for any defects in the material or method of closure. Examine the fluid container for hairline cracks.	Punctures, cracks or any other defects can cause contamination (Goodinson, 1990).
Check the fluid type and the expiry date with the doctor or a second nurse.	For the safety of the patient.
Check the outer wrapper of the administration set is intact before removing.	The wrapper may not withstand wear and tear to which it is subjected — climatic conditions may also affect seals (Goodinson, 1990).
Slide the roller clamp to the top of the tubing next to the drip chamber and close roller clamp.	To prevent air entering the tubing when the infusion fluid is connected to the administration set.
If the clamp is found in the closed position, discard the administration set.	The inside of the administration set is sterilised by free circulation of ethylene oxide gas.
Remove the protective cover from the insertion site of the infusion fluid and the protective cover from the spike of the administration set, taking care to avoid contamination.	To minimise the risk of infection.
Insert the spike into the fluid container. Some administration sets require twisting into position (see manufacturer's instructions).	To pierce the seal.
Hang the infusion onto the drip stand.	

Action	Rationale
Prime the drip chamber by gently squeezing it until half full.	To prevent air entering the tubing.
Remove the cover from the free end of the administration set and lift free end above the level of fluid in the container.	
Open the clamp.	To allow the tubing to be primed with fluid.
Slowly lower the end of the tubing, which will fill with fluid without trapping air.	To prevent air entering the tubing.
Close the clamp.	To prevent fluid escaping from the tubing.
Connect the administration set to the cannula.	To complete the infusion circuit.
Open the clamp.	To allow the infusion to commence.
Regulate the infusion rate in accordance with the patient's prescription chart.	For the safety of the patient and to ensure the fluid is administered at the prescribed rate (Lamb, 1993).
Record in the appropriate documentation.	To maintain an accurate record.

2. Procedure for the care of a patient receiving an intravenous infusion

Action	Rationale
Regulate the drip rate in accordance with the patient's prescription chart, unless using an intravenous fluid pump or controller.	For the safety of the patient.
Record batch number, date and time on the patient's prescription chart and sign.	If any adverse reactions occur, the suspect batch can be identified.
Record all intravenous fluids administered on the fluid balance chart.	To maintain an accurate fluid balance record.
Label the administration set with the date and time of setting up the infusion.	To maintain an accurate record and for the safety of the patient. Administration sets should be changed every 72 hours or after blood transfusion.
Inspect the intravenous site at least daily and prior to giving bolus injections and drugs with a secondary medication system and when changing infusion bags.	To ensure the correct positioning of the cannula and to check for inflammation and/or infection (Lamb, 1993).

Action	Rationale
Check if the patient is experiencing any pain from the infusion.	Inflammation and/or infiltration may cause pain (Lamb, 1993).
Maintain regular temperature recordings.	A mild pyrexia, in the absence of any other clinical signs may be the first indication of infection of the cannula site (Lamb, 1993).
If pain, pyrexia or adverse reactions occur notify the medical staff and stop the infusion immediately.	
N.B. It is advised that the cannula should be resited after a minimum of 72 hours *in situ*.	Incidence of cannula-related sepsis increases after this period of time.
Record in the appropriate documentation.	To maintain an accurate record.

3. Guidelines for the selection of a dressing for the intravenous infusion site

Action	Rationale
The dressing:	
— Must be waterproof, impervious to bacteria and have the ability to keep the skin under the dressing as dry as possible.	Reduces the risk of maceration and reduces the risk of infection associated with excess moisture accumulation.
— Should allow easy visual inspection without removal.	To permit early detection of inflammation, extravasation, collection of blood or pus at insertion site and saves nursing time (Keenlyside, 1992).
— Must be sterile and applied under aseptic conditions (dressings pre-cut to size and sterile are ideal).	Reduces possible contamination through the use of unsterile scissors and tapes (Oldman, 1991).
— Must be easy to apply and conform well to the area of the cannula insertion.	To minimise the risk of the cannula becoming dislodged.
— Must be easy to remove.	To ensure no residual adhesive is left on the skin and the trauma of removing the dressing is minimised.
— Must allow for minimal changes of dressings.	Lowers the risk of introducing bacteria to the venepuncture site and reduces cost.

Action	Rationale
– Must provide secure fixation.	To minimise the risk of the line and cannula dislodging. To minimise any movement of the cannula which could introduce bacteria into the intravascular space and/or cause extravasation of drugs leading to skin breakdown, which would create a potential site for infection (Sheldon, 1994).
– Allow for freedom of movement of the selected limb.	For the comfort and convenience of the patient.
– Apply wound dressing of choice adhering to the appropriate procedure.	To facilitate appropriate application and to maintain asepsis.
– Document the wound dressing on the patient's prescription chart.	In accordance with unit policy for nurses prescribing wound care products.
– Record in the patient's documentation.	To maintain an accurate record.

References

Allwood MC (1981) The control of intravenous infusions. British Journal of Intravenous Therapy 2: (5) 23–5.

Finch RG (1982) Infusion-associated infection — clinical aspects. In D'Arcy PF, (Ed) Infusions and Infections? The Hazards of In-users, Contamination in Intravenous Therapy. Medicine Publishing Symposium Series 6. Oxford: Medicine Publishing Foundation. pp 17–24.

Goodinson SM (1990) Good practice ensures minimum risk factors — Complications of peripheral venous cannulation and infusion therapy. Professional Nurse 6 (3): 175–7.

Hamilton HW, Hamilton KR, Lane FJ (1977) Pre-operative hair removal. Canadian Journal of Surgery 28: 269–74.

Jenner EA (1983) Infuse with safety. Nursing Mirror. April 6: 23–7.

Keenlyside D (1992) Every little detail counts. Infection Control in i.v. therapy. Professional Nurse 7 (4): 226–32.

Lamb J (1993) Peripheral i.v. Therapy. Nursing Standard 7 (36): 31–4.

Muir IFK, Barclay TL (1962) Treatment of burns shock. In Muir IFK, Barclay TL (Eds) Burns and Their Treatment. London: Lloyd-Luke. pp 14–15.

Oldman PA (1991) A sticky solution. A microbiological study of a piece of tape used to secure intravenous cannulae. Professional Nurse. February: 265–9.

Settle JAD (1986) Burns. The First Five Days — Principles of Resuscitation. London: Smith and Nephew Pharmaceuticals pp 13–17.

Sheldon JE (1994) What you should know about i.v. dressings. Nursing 24 (8): 32.

Chapter 17
Care of a patient receiving oxygen therapy

Oxygen therapy is the administration of an increased amount of inspired oxygen in order to allow essential metabolic reactions to occur and to prevent the complications attributed to hypoxaemia.

Indications for oxygen therapy

1. Patients with acute respiratory failure.
2. Patients who require a reduction in ventilatory work in order to maintain oxygenation, e.g. patients with septicaemia.
3. Patients poisoned with carbon monoxide. By increasing arterial oxygen tension, the dissociation of carboxyhaemoglobin is accelerated (Carrougher and Gretchen, 1993).
4. Patients with chronic lung disease.

Hazards of oxygen therapy

1. Oxygen toxicity. Even though oxygen toxicity following exposure to high levels of inspired oxygen is a recognised problem, knowledge of the disorder remains vague.
2. Carbon dioxide narcosis. Administration of more than 28% oxygen to patients with chronic lung disease may lead to a loss of "hypoxic drive". This may lead to severe respiratory failure.

Choice of apparatus and device

1. Ambu bag. This is connected to either the piped oxygen wall supply or an oxygen cylinder. Attached to the bag is either a catheter mount or face mask with an angled connector.
2. Waters bag.
3. Nasal cannulae (see Figure 17.1).
4. Venturi-type masks, e.g. Ventimask (see Figure 17.2).
5. Simple mask, i.e. Hudson (see Figure 17.3).

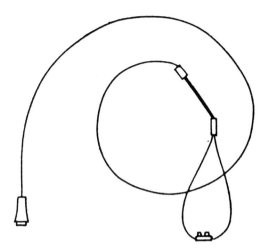

Figure 17.1 *A nasal cannula.*

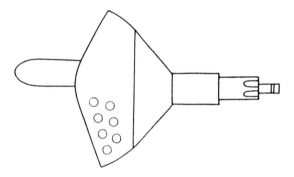

Figure 17.2 *A ventimask.*

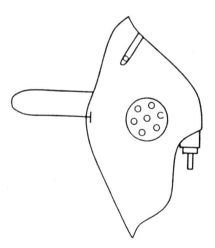

Figure 17.3 *A simple mask.*
(From Mallett and Bailey: The Royal Marsden NHS Trust Manual of Clinical Nursing Procedures 4th Ed (1996) reproduced with permission of Blackwell Science, Oxford.)

1. Procedure for the administration of oxygen therapy

Oxygen therapy is prescribed only by the medical staff (Lancet, 1981).

See sections 2 and 3, this chapter on the administration of humidified oxygen and Chapter 14 on monitoring vital signs. See section 1 in Chapter 1 for advice on procedures.

Equipment

Oxygen supply
Flowmeter
Oxygen bubble tubing
Mask or nasal cannulae

Action	Rationale
Observe and record the patient's vital signs, before, during and after the procedure.	To detect changes in the patient's condition.
Ensure that the patient and relatives are aware of the "no smoking" rule.	Oxygen supports combustion (Allen, 1989).
Measure and record the percentage amount of inspired oxygen.	To ensure the patient is receiving the correct amount of prescribed oxygen.
Position the mask around the patient's face adjusting the straps to fit the face securely. (If the patient has burns to the face, apply paraffin gauze under the straps.)	To ensure the patient receives the correct amount of prescribed oxygen. (Bolgiano, Bunting and Shoenberger, 1990). To maintain patient comfort.
N.B. If using nasal cannulae ensure they are secured well inside the nasal passage.	To ensure the patient receives the correct amount of prescribed oxygen.
Use alternative means of communication.	To prevent the patient constantly removing the mask to speak.
Offer mouth care frequently (or as required).	Oxygen has a drying effect. Mouth care will help to prevent a dry, sore mouth.
Refit the mask regularly.	A loose mask will not deliver the required percentage of oxygen. A tight mask may injure the skin causing sores.
When administering oxygen via nasal cannulae, observe nasal membranes for drying.	At higher flow rates oxygen from nasal cannulae dries the membranes of nostrils.
If the patient is to continue oxygen therapy for over 12 hours refer to the procedure for humidification of oxygen below.	Oxygen is a dry gas and has the potential for drying the mucous membranes of the air passages. Humidified oxygen minimises the risk of dry mucous membranes and is desirable if oxygen therapy is to be continued for long periods of time.
Record in the appropriate documentation.	To maintain an accurate record.

2. Care of a patient receiving humidified oxygen therapy

Normally the function of the upper airway is to warm, moisten and filter inspired gases. As a result of disease processes and/or inhalation injuries in burns patients, these functions are impaired and additional humidification may be required. Humidification increases the moisture content of inspired gases and assists/replaces the function of the upper airway.

Indications

Humidification is nearly always required for self-ventilating patients requiring oxygen therapy.

1. It facilitates expectoration.
2. It minimises the possibility of sputum retention.
3. It allows clearing of secretions from the respiratory tree.
4. It prevents increased mucous viscosity with crusting, tracheal inflammation and mucosal ulceration.

Contraindications

Humidified oxygen therapy is contraindicated in the following situations.

1. Acute and severe pulmonary oedema where the aspirate is watery. If the aspirate is heavily bloodstained humidification may be required to prevent clotting in the larger airways.
2. Intermittent high flow therapy for physiotherapy, where the therapy is only instituted for a short time.

Complications

1. Infection (water reservoirs have frequently grown pseudomonas aeruginosa).
2. Overhydration.
3. Hyperpyrexia as a result of constantly elevated inspired gases.
4. Tracheal scalding.
5. Electrical hazards.

Types of humidification devices

1. Hot water bath humidifiers (see Figure 17.4)
2. Nebulizers. These devices deliver micro-droplets of water suspended in a gaseous medium, e.g. ultrasonic.
3. Individual water pack systems (for temporary use only as they may be unreliable). (See Figure 17.5).

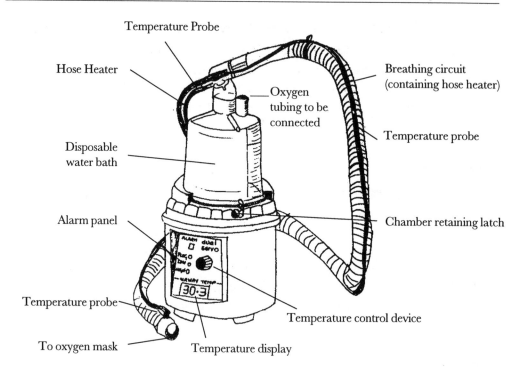

Figure 17.4 *A hot water bath humidifier.*

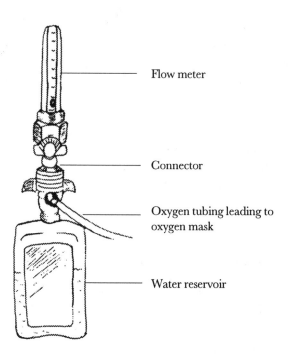

Figure 17.5 *An individual water pack system.*

3. Procedure for the administration of humidified oxygen

Oxygen therapy is prescribed only by the medical staff.

See section on nursing procedures for administration of oxygen above and section 1 in Chapter 1 for advice on procedures.

Equipment

Oxygen supply. This may be a piped supply or from a portable cylinder

Flowmeter tubing. This may be green bubble tubing which is used only in the short term, as humidification is not required. Larger diameter corrugated tubing is required for the administration of humidified oxygen

Delivery mechanism, e.g. mask or cannula

Humidifier

Sterile water (or individual water pack system for temporary use)

Oxygen analyser

Action	Rationale
Ensure the humidification apparatus features safety mechanisms against overheating, over-hydration and electrocution.	For the safety of the patient (Chamney, 1969).
Place the oxygen analyser on the input side of the humidifer	To prevent condensation within the analyser causing errors when reading.
Position the humidifer below the level of the oxygen mask.	To prevent "drowning" with condensed water.
Check the temperature controls of the system every hour.	To ensure the humidifier machine is operating at the intended temperature.
Ensure the delivered oxygen is between 23° C and 37° C.	To ensure maximum water content of the inspired oxygen. To prevent scalding of the trachea.
Fill the water bath with sterile water.	To reduce the risk of transferring infection (Rhame et al., 1986).
Check the water level of the bath frequently and top up as necessary.	To maintain adequate humidification.
Never empty condensed water back into the water bath.	To prevent colonisation of the bath with potential pathogens.
Immediately clear away all spilt water or condensation.	To prevent electrical injury.
Change the water bath tubing every 24–48 hours.	To prevent colonisation of pseudomonas aeruginosa infection (Rhame et al., 1986).

Action	Rationale
Record the percentage of oxygen being delivered in the appropriate documentation.	To maintain an accurate record.

References

Allen D (1989) Making sense of oxygen delivery. Nursing Times 85 (18): 40–2.

Bolgiano CS, Bunting K, Shoenberger MM (1990) Administering oxygen therapy. What you need to know. Nursing 20: 47–51.

Carrougher CJ, Gretchen J (1993) Inhalation injury. American Association of Clinical Nursing – Clinical Issues 4 (2): 367–76.

Chamney AR (1969) Humidification requirements and techniques. Anaesthesia 24: 602–17.

Lancet (1981) Acute oxygen therapy. Lancet 1: 980–1.

Rhame FS, Streifel A, McComb C, Boyle M (1986) Bubbling humidifiers produce microaerosis which can carry bacteria. Infection Control 7: 403–7.

Further Reading

Health Equipment Information (1986) 151, January, NHS Procurement Directorate.

Health Equipment Information (1987) 177, January, NHS Procurement Directorate.

Martin K (1991) Oxygen delivery and consumption in septic shock. Intensive Care Nursing 7 (4): 193–9.

Oh TE (1990) Intensive Care Manual (3rd Edition) London: Butterworths. pp 128–33.

Chapter 18
Care of a patient with an arterial line

An arterial line is a percutaneous cannula placed within an artery. It is kept patent by a continuous infusion of heparinised saline via a pressurised flushing device (see Figure 18.1).

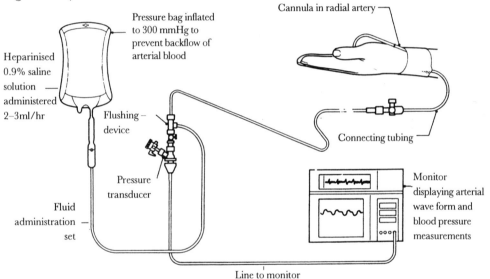

Figure 18.1 *Arterial blood pressure monitoring system.*
Adapted from Wilkie A.V (1992) Blood pressure monitoring. Surgical Nurse 5–(2): 18–22

Indications

Any critically ill burns trauma patient whose respiratory function is compromised will require an arterial line, which is used for:

1. Repeated blood sampling.
2. Continuous monitoring of blood pressure.

Sites for insertion (Low, 1990)

1. Radial artery (most commonly used).
2. Dorsalis pedis.

3. Brachial artery.
4. Axillary artery.
5. Femoral artery.

Complications

Haemorrhage
1. Locally at the site.
2. Following removal of the cannula.
3. Due to accidental disconnection.

Infection
1. Locally at the site.
2. Septicaemia

Thrombus formation at the tip of the cannula.
Embolism
1. Air.
2. Clot.
3. Septic.

Ischaemia of the limb distal to the cannula.
Pain or loss of sensation due to nerve damage.
Haematoma at the site of insertion.
Arterial spasm on manual flushing of the line.

1. Procedure for the care of a patient undergoing arterial cannulation

Arterial cannulae are inserted only by medical staff.
See sections 1–5 in Chapter 1 for advice on procedures and sharps policy.

Equipment

Trolley
Sterile dressing pack
Skin antiseptic solution. 10% Povidone Iodine with alcohol or Chlorhexadine
    0.5% (red) with alcohol
Arterial cannulae (of choice)
Sterile semi-permeable film dressing
Local anaesthetic agent
Sterile needle and syringe
1 pair of sterile gloves
Hand held suture

An arterial line administration set connected to a 500 ml pressurised bag of
    heparinised 0.9% saline (500 ml)
Pressure bag
Sharps box

Action	Rationale
Expose the site to be cannulated.	To allow access to the artery/insertion site.
The doctor	
– Cleans the site with the skin antiseptic solution of choice.	To maintain asepsis.
– Instils the local anaesthetic into the skin.	To minimise pain and discomfort during the procedure (Sprung and Grenvik, 1985).
– Inserts the arterial cannula.	To provide arterial access.
– Sutures the cannula to the skin.	To secure the cannula in position.
Connect the administration set to the cannula.	To provide a continuous flushing device to maintain patency of the cannula.
Flush the cannula.	To confirm that the cannula is patent.
Apply the semi-permeable film dressing over the cannula insertion site.	To allow easy viewing of the insertion site. To protect the wound from contamination and to secure the cannula in position (Mughal and Leinhardt, 1990).
Ensure the arterial line is visible at all times.	To minimise the risk of disconnection or dislodgement.
Inflate the pressure bag to 300 mmHg.	To maintain cannula patency via the flushing device.
Maintain frequent observation of the catheter. Avoid any traction on the line and keep the line visible if possible.	To prevent dislodgement or disconnection that could result in a major arterial haemorrhage (Allen, 1990).
Dispose of the sharps into the sharps box.	In accordance with unit sharps policy, to prevent needlestick injuries.
Record in the appropriate documentation.	To maintain an accurate record.

2. Procedure for taking an arterial blood gas specimen from an arterial line

See sections 1, 2, 3, and 5 in Chapter 1 for advice on procedures and sharps policy.

Equipment

1 pair of unsterile gloves
Cardboard tray/receiver
Alcohol wipe
Sterile non-injectable luer lock cap
1 needle
2 x 2 ml syringes
Heparin (1000 units/ml)
Blind hub
Sharps box

Action	Rationale
Using the needle, draw back 1 ml of heparin into a 2 ml syringe. Shake the syringe to coat the inside of the barrel, expel heparin from syringe.	To provide anticoagulant for the blood specimen.
Apply unsterile gloves.	To protect the nurse from blood-borne infections.
Remove the cap from the three-way tap proximal to patient.	To provide access for removal of blood.
Clean the port with the alcohol-based wipe and allow to air dry.	To maintain asepsis.
Insert the non-heparinised syringe into the port and turn the three-way tap so that blood flows from the patient into the syringe. Withdraw 2 ml of blood.	To clear the line of heparinised saline.
Turn the tap 45°.	To occlude flow from and to the patient.
Remove the blood-filled syringe and place in the cardboard tray/receiver (discard).	To prevent blood spillage.
Insert the heparinised syringe into the port, turn the three-way tap 45° and withdraw 1 ml of blood.	To obtain the sample.
Turn the tap 90° and remove the syringe, cover the port with the blind hub and place the blood-filled syringe in the cardboard tray/receiver.	To prevent blood spillage and specimen contamination.
Flush the blood remaining in the line into the patient using the manual flush device.	To clear the line of residual blood.

Action	Rationale
Turn the tap 90° so that flow to and from the artery is occluded and flush blood from the three-way tap into the cardboard tray/receiver.	To clear the tap of residual blood.
Turn the tap 90° so that the entry port is occluded.	To allow a continuous flow of heparinised saline through the arterial cannula.
Place the sterile luer lock cap on the port.	To prevent blood leakage and contamination.
Place all sharps into sharps box, discard all used equipment and remove gloves.	According to unit sharps policy and to prevent cross infection with blood-borne organisms.
Record the patient's temperature, the current percentage of oxygen being delivered and the present haemoglobin level and send this information with the sample.	The blood gas analyser machine calibrates the results of the sample according to these variables.
Immediately take the blood-filled syringe for analysis.	To prevent the blood from clotting.
Following analysis of the sample, record the results in the appropriate documentation.	To maintain an accurate record.

References

Allen D (1989) Making sense of arterial catheterisation. Nursing Times 85 (40): 45–7.
Low JM (1990) Haemodynamic monitoring. In: Oh TE, (Ed) Intensive Care Manual (3rd Edition) Sydney: Butterworths.
Mughal M, Leinhardt A (1990) Infected feeding lines. Care of the Critically Ill 6: 228–32.
Sprung CL, Grenvik A (1985) Invasive Procedures in Critical Care. Edinburgh: Churchill Livingstone.

Further Reading

Rainbow C (1989) Monitoring the critically ill patient. Heinemann Nursing.
Wilkie AV (1992) Blood pressure monitoring. Surgical Nurse 5 (2): 18–22.

Chapter 19
Care of a patient with a tracheostomy

A tracheostomy is an artificial opening in the trachea into which a tube is inserted (see Figures 19.1 and 19.2). Air enters via the stoma, bypassing the normal filtering, moistening and warming functions performed by the nasal mucosa.

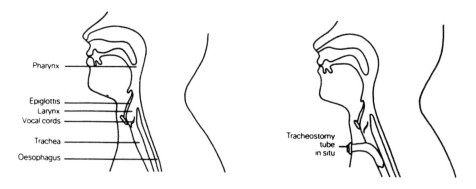

Figure 19.1 *Anatomy of the head and neck.*   Figure 19.2 *Tracheostomy.*
(From Mallett and Bailey: Royal Marsden Hospital NHS Trust Manual of Clinical Nursing Procedures 4th Ed (1996) reproduced with permission of Blackwell Science, Oxford)

Indications for tracheostomy (Heffner, Miller and Sahn, 1986 a,b)

1. To improve pulmonary hygiene/bronchial toilet.
2. For the relief of upper airway obstruction.
3. For long-term mechanical ventilation. At the first sign of impending airway obstruction following a burn injury, control of the upper airway is achieved by either endotracheal intubation or tracheostomy (Herndon, Thompson and Traber, 1985). This includes patients who present with stridor, dyspnoea, respiratory depression, pharyngeal swelling, nasolabial full thickness burns, circumferential neck burns and burns of the upper airway (Bartlett et al., 1976; Bayley, 1991).
4. In patients who are difficult to wean from the ventilator.

Complications

1. Apnoea and hypertension. Control of the upper airway is achieved by either endotracheal intubation or tracheostomy at the first sign of impending airway obstruction following a burn injury (Herndon, Thompson and Traber, 1985). This includes patients who present with stridor, dyspnoea, respiratory depression, pharyngeal swelling, nasolabial full thickness burns, circumferential neck burns and burns of the upper airway (Bartlett et al., 1976; Bayley, 1991).
   The administration of either artificial respiration or 5% carbon dioxide may be necessary for some hours until the patient starts breathing again. The sudden decrease in carbon dioxide level may also lead to hypertension.
2. Haemorrhage. During the procedure haemorrhage may occur from the anterior jugular system, from the thyroid isthmus or from the tracheal wall. Secondary haemorrhage may occur as a result of infection around the stoma site. Fatal erosion of a large artery can occur from ulceration of the anterior wall of the trachea by pressure of the tip of an incorrectly fitting tracheostomy.
3. Damage to the oesophagus. If the trachea is incised during inspiration, the wall of the oesophagus may be drawn forward and damaged.
4. Damage to the cricoid cartilage. If the tracheostomy is established in the first or second tracheal rings, chondritis of the cricoid cartilage may occur. The cartilage collapses causing the airway to become permanently useless.
5. Pulmonary infection (Harris and Hyman, 1984). This occurs as a result of:
   - Unsterile suction technique (Landis and McLane, 1979).
   - Incorrect length of tracheostomy tube.
   - "Self infection" as a result of a back flow of gastric/oesophageal secretions into the trachea.
   - Colonisation of the tracheostomy tube by micro-organisms (around the tracheostomy site and then tracking downwards).
6. Surgical emphysema. Occurs as a result of overtight suturing of the tracheostomy wound.
7. Displacement of the tube into the pretracheal space caused by either insecure tying of the tube around the neck or rapid cervical swelling.
8. Tracheal stenosis.
9. Dysphagia.
10. Failure of closure of the fistula after removal of the tube.
11. Pneumothorax.

Types of tracheostomy

1. Elective temporary tracheostomy.
2. Permanent tracheostomy.
3. Emergency tracheostomy.

Types of tracheostomy tube (Weilitz and Dettenmeier, 1994)

1. Portex cuffed tracheostomy tube (see Figure 19.3). A disposable tube with an introducer.
2. Portex uncuffed tracheostomy tube (see Figure 19.4).

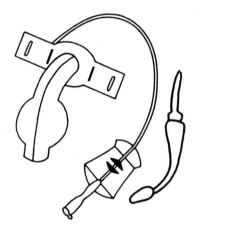

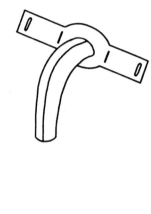

Figure 19.3 *A Portex cuffed tube.*   Figure 19.4 *A Portex uncuffed tube.*

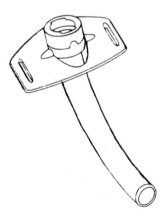

Figure 19.5 *A Shiley cuffless tracheostomy tube.*

3. Shiley cuffless tracheostomy tube. For long-term or permanent tracheostomy patients who do not require ventilation (see Figure 19.5).
4. Shiley low pressure cuffed tracheostomy tube. Allows safe and effective ventilation, whilst minimising the possibility of tracheal wall damage (see Figure 19.6).
5. Shiley fenestrated low pressure cuffed tracheostomy tube. Allows effective weaning from the ventilator. This is a plastic tube with an introducer and two inner tubes.

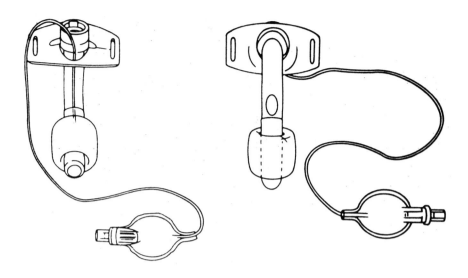

Figure 19.6 *A Shiley low pressure cuffed tracheostomy tube.*

6. Shiley plain fenestrated tube. This is a plastic device with a two-way valve which fits onto the Shiley inner tube (see Figure 19.7).

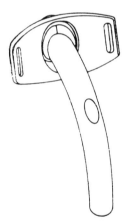

Figure 19.7 *A Shiley plain fenestrated tube.*

7. Silver tracheostomy tube. This is a silver tube with an introducer and two inner tubes with or without speaking valves (see Figure 19.8).

1. Procedure for the post-operative care of a patient with a tracheostomy

See section 7 in this chapter on caring for a patient undergoing tracheal suction, Chapter 14 for advice on monitoring vital signs, and section 1, Chapter 1 for advice on procedures.

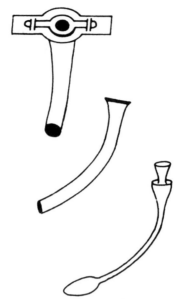

Figure 19.8 *A silver tube.*
(Figures 19.3–19.8 *from Mallett and Bailey: Royal Marsden Hospital NHS Trust Manual of Clinical Nursing Procedures 4th Ed (1996) reproduced with permission of Blackwell Science, Oxford.*)

Equipment

Humidifier
Oxygen supply, T-piece and oxygen tubing
Suction equipment
Suction catheters
Sterile disposable gloves
Water for rinsing suction tubing
Writing equipment, word boards
Tracheal dilators
A selection of different sized tracheostomy tubes (one portex — smaller size)
Lubricating gel
Sterile tracheostomy dressing (optional)

Action	Rationale
Ensure the patient is placed in a semiprone position.	To ensure a clear airway. To facilitate respiration, promote drainage, minimise oedema and prevent strain on the suture line.
Record the patient's vital signs. Administer prescribed oxygen.	To detect any changes in the patient's condition.
Provide humidification for oxygen therapy.	To prevent accumulation of dry secretions (Oh, 1990).
Ensure adequate fixation of the tracheostomy tube.	To prevent displacement of the tube.

Action	Rationale
N.B. It is essential not to tie the tapes too loose or too tight, and aim to keep the head flexed.	The tapes secure the tube in position. To prevent discomfort for the patient and to relax the neck muscles.
Administer tracheal suction as required.	To maintain a clear airway.
Perform mouth care as required.	To maintain oral cleanliness. To promote patient comfort.
Assist with the chest X-ray.	To establish the position of the tube and to exclude pneumothorax.
Record in the appropriate nursing documentation.	To maintain an accurate record.

2. Procedure for the care of a patient requiring tracheal suction via a tracheostomy tube

Patients with an artificial airway are unable to cough and expectorate effectively, therefore tracheal secretions are removed by tracheal suction.

Complications

1. Hypoxaemia. During suction, oxygen enriched air is sucked out of the lungs. This may cause severe hypoxaemia and bradycardia.
2. Cardiac dysrhythmias. These may occur as a result of arterial and thus myocardial hypoxia or as a result of vagal stimulation secondary to tracheal irritation.
3. Hypotension may occur due to profound bradycardia or prolonged coughing during the procedure.
4. Alveolar collapse.
5. Tracheal mucosal damage.
6. Secondary pulmonary infection.
7. Raised intracranial pressure.

In patients with impaired/unstable neurological function, suctioning may increase intracranial pressure above normal limits. This may occur as a result of the raised intrathoracic pressure associated with coughing.

See sections 1 and 5 in Chapter 1 for advice on procedures.

Equipment

Suction catheters — the catheter diameter should be half the diameter of the endotracheal tube, e.g. for a 7 mm endotracheal tube use a 14 (fg) catheter (Allen, 1988).

Vacuum supply/suction unit

Collection system
Suction tubing
1 pair of sterile gloves
Water for cleaning suction tubing
Specimen trap
Extra-long suction catheters

Action	Rationale
Assess for the presence of secretions: – Tachycardia – Reduced oxygen saturation – Bubbling noises during inspiration – Reduced air entry – Crackles on auscultation Monitor and assess: – Cardiovascular status – Respiratory status – Consciousness level	To assess the need for suctioning (Allen, 1988).
Encourage the patient to take a deep breath in and cough if able.	To give the patient the chance to loosen and clear his or her own secretions.
Explain the procedure to the patient.	Provides psychological support (Glandis and McLance, 1979).
Pre-oxygenate the patient (if required).	To prevent hypoxaemia and bradycardia (Barnes and Kirchoff, 1986; Brown et al., 1983).
Switch on suction unit to desired level according to the age of the patient ensuring it does not exceed 100–150 mmHg.	If the suction is set too high it may damage the trachea, if it is too low it will be ineffective (Allen, 1988).
Open the top of the sterile catheter to expose the hub without removing the wrapper.	To maintain asepsis (Harris and Hyman, 1984).
Attach the specimen trap (if tracheal aspirate specimen is required).	Sputum specimens may be sent for culture if a chest infection is suspected.
Connect the hub to the suction tubing.	
Avoiding contamination, partially withdraw the catheter from the sleeve.	To maintain asepsis.
Apply sterile gloves.	Gloves minimise the risk of cross infection.
Withdraw the remaining length of the catheter.	
At the end of a complete inspiratory phase, remove oxygen tubing and place it on the sterile glove cover.	To ensure optimal oxygenation prior to suction. To minimise the risk of cross infection.

Action	Rationale
Insert the catheter into the airway until resistance is felt.	
Encourage the patient to cough or apply chest vibrations.	To aid elimination of secretions.
Withdraw the catheter approximately 1 cm with suction off.	To avoid damage to the carina.
Apply intermittent suction by occluding the hole on hub as the catheter is withdrawn, using a rotating action. Do not suction the patient for longer than 10–15 seconds.	To remove secretions around the mucous membranes (Allen, 1988). To prevent alveolar collapse, hypoxia and a choking sensation for the patient.
Withdraw the catheter from the trachea having released the thumb from the hub.	To release suction and prevent trauma to the tracheal mucosa.
Reconnect the patient to the oxygen supply (with clean hand).	To maintain oxygen therapy and reduce the risk of desaturation (Brown et al., 1983).
Assess the amount and type of secretions and whether the procedure needs to be repeated.	To assess the effectiveness of suction.
Wrap the catheter in the glove and discard.	To minimise the risk of cross infection.
Rinse the connection tubing by suctioning the water.	To remove secretions which have adhered to the inside of the tubing.
Turn off suction apparatus.	
Label all specimens and send to the microbiology laboratory.	For appropriate investigations to be carried out.
Record amount, type, colour and consistency of secretions in the appropriate documentation.	To maintain an accurate record.

3. Procedure for changing a tracheostomy dressing

This procedure requires two nurses. Facilities for emergency intubation must be available in case of accidental removal of the tube.

See section 2, this chapter for the procedure for caring for a patient undergoing tracheal suction and sections 1–5 in Chapter 1 for advice on procedures.

Equipment

Trolley
Sterile dressing pack
1 pair of sterile gloves
1 pair of unsterile gloves

Sterile scissors
Sterile tracheostomy dressing (of choice)
Sachet of saline and alcohol swab
Alcohol-based hand wash solution
Tracheostomy tapes

Action	Rationale
Suction the airway.	When the dressing is loosened most patients cough and produce secretions which have adhered to the inside of the tube.
Nurse One:	
– Apply unsterile gloves, remove and discard the soiled dressing.	To minimise the risk of cross infection. To avoid patient discomfort.
– Removed soiled tapes.	To change the tapes and to prevent displacement of the tube.
– Nurse one to hold the tracheostomy in place.	
Nurse Two:	
– Apply sterile gloves	
– If exudate is present, clean the skin with sterile saline.	To remove exudate and to minimise the risk of cross infection.
– Assess the wound for redness, swelling, oozing, odour and inflammation.	To observe signs of complications.
– Apply the sterile tracheostomy dressing of choice, except gauze.	To maintain patient comfort (avoid pressure). Gauze may shed filaments and they will lodge in the stoma (Caruana, 1990).
– Secure the tube with clean tapes.	To prevent dislodgement of the tube.
Both nurses:	
Tie the tapes with a reef-knot (not in a bow).	To prevent untying of the knot (De Clarle, 1985).
Remove gloves and wash hands.	
Ensure the patient is left in a comfortable position.	For the comfort of the patient.
Record in the appropriate nursing documentation.	To maintain an accurate record.

4. Procedure for changing a tracheostomy tube

The medical staff should perform the first tracheostomy change (usually after 5 days). The sutures are usually removed during the first change. A nurse may perform subsequent changes every 7 days. It is advisable to ensure a member of the medical staff is present on the unit at the time of the change.

Changing the tube

This is a two-nurse procedure. Facilities for emergency intubation should be available in case of a difficult tube change as a result of an unpredicted shape or angle of the stoma or tracheal stenosis.

See section 2, this chapter on caring for a patient undergoing tracheal suction, and sections 1–5 in Chapter 1 for advice on procedures and sharps policy.

Equipment

Trolley
Sterile dressing pack
Sterile tracheostomy dressing (of choice)
Tracheostomy tubes, one the same size and one a size smaller
Tracheostomy tapes
1 pair of sterile gloves
1 pair of unsterile gloves
Sachet of saline and alcohol swab
Sterile gauze swabs
Lubricating gel
10 ml syringe
Stitch cutter
Suction equipment
Tracheal dilators
Cuff pressure gauge
Sharps box

Action	Rationale
Position the patient as flat as their condition allows.	To hyperextend the neck; skin folds may occlude the site.
Pre-oxygenate the patient if necessary. Nurse One:	To prevent hypoxia (Barnes and Kirchoff, 1986).
– Apply sterile gloves.	To maintain asepsis. The tube is difficult to manipulate with forceps.
– Place the tracheostomy tapes through the slits in the flanges.	To allow easier fixation of the tubes.
– Place the dressing in advance around the new tube.	To prevent abrasion of the patient's skin by the tube.

Action	Rationale
– Fully inflate and deflate the cuff.	To avoid insertion of a faulty tube.
– Place the introducer in position.	To allow easier passage of the tube along the contour of the trachea.
– Lubricate the tube.	To facilitate introducing the tube into the trachea.
Nurse Two:	
– Suction the trachea.	To prevent additional coughing. To minimise secretions during the change.
– Deflate the cuff on the old tube.	To prevent traumatic removal of the tube.
– Apply unsterile gloves and cut the tapes around the patient's neck.	To facilitate removal of the tube.
– Remove the soiled dressing and tube whilst asking the patient to breathe out.	Expiration reduces the risk of coughing.
Nurse One:	
– If exudate is present, clean around the stoma site with the saline and dry gently using the sterile gauze swabs.	To remove superficial micro-organisms.
Insert the clean tube using an up and over action.	To introduce the tube along the contour of the trachea.
Remove the introducer.	
Inflate the cuff.	To secure the tube. To prevent aspiration of secretions.
Check the patient can breathe out of the tube.	To ensure that the tube is in the correct position.
Apply the sterile tracheostomy dressing of choice.	To maintain patient comfort.
Remove gloves and wash hands.	To minimise the risk of infection.
Assist Nurse Two in tying the tapes around the neck in a reefknot.	To secure the tube in position and prevent untying of the knot (De Clarle, 1985).
Ensure the patient is left in a comfortable position.	To maintain patient safety.
Observe the patient for complications.	To maintain patient safety.
Record in the appropriate nursing documentation.	To maintain an accurate record.

5. Procedure for the care of a patient with a minitracheostomy

Minitracheostomy involves the insertion of a fine bore tube through the cricothyroid membrane into the trachea to allow aspiration of retained secretions from the tracheobronchial tree, thereby preventing sputum retention.

Indications for minitracheostomy

1. Sputum retention (Mathews and Hopkinson, 1984).
2. Emergency provision and maintenance of airway.
3. Artificial ventilation.
4. Jet ventilation to facilitate bronchial toilet (Frame, Eve and Walker, 1986).
5. Oxygen administration.

Contraindications

1. Respiratory failure due to loss of respiratory drive or lung function. Insertion of a minitracheostomy under these circumstances is not therapeutic, and potentially dangerous.
2. Children under the age of 12 years (Frame, Eve and Walker, 1986).

Complications of insertion of a minitracheostomy

1. Haemorrhage.
2. Pneumothorax.
3. Laryngeal stricture (subglottic stenosis).
4. Bronchospasm.
5. Tube malposition.
6. Local or systemic infection.
7. Surgical emphysema.
8. Loss of the tube in the trachea (Yeoh, Wells and Goldstraw, 1985) (a particular risk when a split paediatric endotracheal tube is used).

6. Procedure for the insertion of a minitracheostomy tube

Minitracheostomy insertion is performed only by medical staff. The procedure is safe and easily performed (Kirk, 1986; Matthews and Hopkinson, 1984). It provides ready access to main airways for lavage and suction, and there is no interference with speech, ventilation or swallowing. After removal of the minitracheostomy tube the fistula heals quickly with an acceptable cosmetic scar. There is no evidence of tracheal stenosis following the procedure (Frame, Eve and Walker, 1986).

Venous access and facilities for emergency intubation and artificial ventilation must be available. Suction equipment with a Y-connector and a 10 (fg) suction catheter must be available and working at the bedside.

See sections 1–5 in Chapter 1 for advice on procedures and sharps policy.

Equipment

Trolley
Sterile dressing pack
Skin antiseptic solution, e.g. 10% Povidone Iodine with alcohol or Chlorhexidine
0.5% (red) with alcohol
Skin anaesthetic
Selection of syringes and needles
1 pair of sterile gloves
Sharps box
Minitracheostomy kit containing:
  Introducer
  Scalpel
  Suture
  Tube
  Tape
  10 (fg) suction catheter
  15 mm connector

Action	Rationale
Position the patient as requested by the doctor. Usual positions are either lying flat or sitting slightly upright with the neck slightly extended.	To allow location and palpation of the trachea.
Expose the patient's neck.	To allow access to the insertion site.
The doctor:	
– Applies sterile gloves.	To maintain asepsis.
– Cleans the skin with the antiseptic solution of choice.	To minimise the risk of infection.
– Instils local anaesthetic into the skin.	To minimise pain and discomfort during the procedure.
– Makes a small incision with a scalpel.	To facilitate insertion of the tube through the tracheal wall.
– Inserts the minitracheostomy tube.	
– Removes the introducer from the lumen of the minitracheostomy tube.	To check the position of the tube and to ensure its patency.
– Applies suction via the minitracheostomy with the catheter provided.	To clear accumulated secretions and blood from the site of tube insertion.
– Sutures the minitracheostomy tube in position.	To ensure a good position and prevent accidental removal (Yeoh, Wells and Goldstraw, 1985).

Action	Rationale
– Inserts the tapes through the flanges of the tube and secures them around the patient's neck. Observe and record the patient's respiratory rate as requested by the medical staff. Assist the radiographer with a chest X-ray. Record in the appropriate nursing documentation.	Respiratory distress and bronchospasm may occur. To check the position of the minitracheostomy. To maintain an accurate record.

7. Procedure for tracheal suction via a minitracheostomy

See section 2, this chapter for advice on caring for a patient undergoing tracheal suction and sections 1 and 2 in Chapter 1 for advice on procedures.

Equipment

Vacuum supply/suction unit
Collection system
Suction tubing
1 pair of sterile gloves
Water for cleaning suction tubing
Y-connector
10 (fg) and 8 (fg) suction catheters

Action	Rationale
Assess for the presence of:	To assess the need for suctioning.
– Secretions. – Tachycardia. – Reduced oxygen saturation. – Bubbling noises during inspiration. – Reduced air entry.	
Monitor and assess:	
– Cardiovascular status. – Respiratory status. – Consciousness level.	To assess the patient's general condition prior to performing the procedure.
Pre-oxygenate the patient (if required).	To prevent hypoxaemia and bradycardia.
Switch on suction unit to desired level according to the age of the patient.	
Open the top of the sterile catheter to expose	

Action	Rationale
Open the top of the sterile catheter to expose the hub.	To maintain asepsis.
Attach the specimen trap (if tracheal aspirate specimen is required).	To obtain a specimen for investigation.
Connect the hub to the suction tubing via a Y-connector.	To provide a way of regulating the pressures.
Avoiding contamination, partially withdraw the catheter from the sleeve.	To maintain asepsis.
Apply sterile gloves.	Gloves minimise the risk of cross infection.
Withdraw the remaining length of catheter.	
Using the clean hand remove the minitracheostomy cap.	To provide access to the airway.
Insert the catheter into the airway until resistance is felt.	
Encourage the patient to cough or apply chest vibrations.	To aid elimination of secretions.
Withdraw the catheter approximately 1 cm with suction off.	To avoid damage to the carina.
Apply intermittent suction by occluding the hole on the hub of the Y-connector.	The patient continues to breathe through the nose and mouth because the minitracheostomy only partially occludes the trachea.
If possible leave the catheter in position for the duration of the physiotherapy.	The benefits of chest physiotherapy may be maximised.
Withdraw the catheter from the trachea having released thumb from the hub.	To release suction and prevent trauma to the tracheal mucosa.
Close the minitracheostomy cap.	
Assess the amount and type of secretions.	To assess effectiveness of suction.
Wrap the catheter in the glove and discard.	To minimise the risk of cross infection.
Rinse the connection tubing by suctioning the water.	To remove secretions which have adhered to the inside of the tubing.
Turn off suction apparatus.	
Label any specimens and send to the microbiology laboratory.	For appropriate investigations to be carried out.
Record amount, type, colour, and consistency of secretions in the appropriate documentation.	To maintain an accurate record.

References

Allen D (1988) Making sense of suctioning. Nursing Times 84 (10): 46–7.

Barnes CA, Kirchoff KT (1986) Minimising hypoxaemia due to endotracheal suctioning. A review of the literature. Heart and Lung 15 (2): 164–76.

Bartlett RH et al. (1976) Acute management of the upper airway in facial burns. Archives of Surgery 111: 744.

Bayley EW (1991) Care of the burn patient with an inhalation injury. In Trofino RB, (Ed) Nursing Care of the Burn Injured Patient. Philadelphia: FA Davis. pp 333–4.

Brown SE, Stansbury DW, Merill E, Linden MD, Light RW (1983) Prevention of suction related oxygen desaturation. Chest 83 (4): 621–7.

Caruana SR (1990) Myths and facts about tracheal tubes. Nursing (US) 5 (11): 66–72.

De Clarle B (1985) Tracheostomy care. Nursing Times (occasional paper) 8.1 (40): 54–60.

Frame JD, Eve MD, Walker CC (1986) The use of minitracheostomy technique in burned patients. Burns Journal 12: 440–2.

Glandis J, McLance AM (1979) Tracheal suctioning: a tool for evaluation and learning needs assessment. Nursing Research 28 (4): 237–42.

Harris RB, Hyman RB (1984) Clean vs sterile tracheostomy care and level of pulmonary infection. Nursing Research 33 (2): 80–4.

Heffner JE, Miller S, Sahn SA (1986a) Tracheostomy in the intensive care unit. Part 1: Indications, technique, management. Chest 90 (2): 269–74.

Heffner JE, Miller S, Sahn SA (1986b) Tracheostomy in the intensive care unit. Part 2: Complications. Chest 90 (3): 430–6.

Herndon DN, Thompson PB, Traber DL (1985) Pulmonary injury in burned patients. Proceedings of the Symposium: Respiratory Care of the Burned Patient. Orlando Florida: American Burn Association. p 15.

Kirk AJB (1986) Minitracheostomy in cardiothoracic practice. Care of the Critically Ill 2 (3): 104–10.

Landis IG, McLane A (1979) Tracheal suctioning a tool for evaluation and learning needs assessment. Nursing Research 28: 237–42.

Matthews HR, Hopkinson RB (1984) Treatment of sputum retention by mini-tracheostomy. British Journal of Surgery 71: 147.

Oh TE (1990) Intensive Care Manual. London: Butterworths. pp 169–73.

Weilitz PB, Dettenmeier PA (1994) Test your knowledge of tracheostomy tubes. American Journal of Nursing. February: 46–50.

Yeoh NTL, Wells FC, Goldstraw P (1985) A complication of mini-tracheostomy. British Journal of Surgery 72: 633.

Further Reading

Iveson T (1981) Student's Forum. Tracheostomy, Nursing Mirror. Volume 153, Number 4, pp 30–1.

Johnson BC, Wells ST, Dungca CU, Hoffmeister D (1988) Standards of Critical Care. p 36–40 CV Mosby Company.

Matthews HR et al. (1986) Minitracheostomy — A delivery system for jet ventilation. Journal of Thoracic and Cardiothoracic Surgery 2: 673–5.

Nursing US (1976) Up to Date Survey of Tracheal Tubes. Nursing (US) Volume 5, Number 11 pp 66–72.

Chapter 20
Care of a patient with a central venous catheter

Central venous catheterisation involves percutaneous insertion of a hollow, radio-opaque cannula, the tip of which lies either in the right atrium or in the superior vena cava (see Figure 20.1).

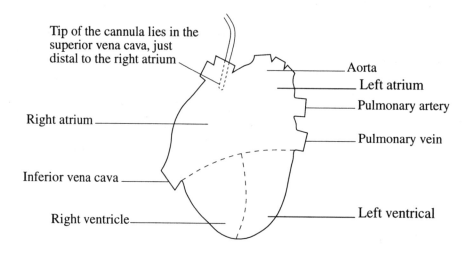

Tip of the cannula lies in the superior vena cava, just distal to the right atrium

Aorta
Left atrium
Pulmonary artery

Right atrium

Pulmonary vein

Inferior vena cava

Right ventricle

Left ventrical

Figure 20.1 *The site and position of a central venous catheter.*

Indications

Central venous catheterisation allows rapid infusion of high volumes of fluids, e.g. during the fluid resuscitation of a patient in shock or following major burns surgery. It facilitates assessment of the patient's haemodynamic status. Measurement of the central venous pressure (i.e. the pressure in the right atrium) gives information about right-sided heart function and intravascular fluid volume. It allows infusion of drugs and fluids which are venous irritants, e.g. dopamine and hypertonic dextrose solutions, the infusion of which via peripheral veins may cause inflammation and necrosis. Lastly, it allows long-term parenteral nutrition while minimising potential hazards, e.g. venous drainage and septicaemia.

Contraindications

Pre-existing infection of the puncture site. A patient on a full anticoagulation regime is in danger of bleeding from puncture sites and the potential benefits of central venous catheterisation must be weighed against possible risks.

Complications

1. During insertion:
   - Introduction of infection.
   - Pneumothorax.
   - Misplacement of the cannula, e.g. in the right ventricle, or threading up the neck veins from a subclavian approach.
   - Pain and discomfort for the patient.
   - Arrhythmias.
   - Air embolism.
2. Post insertion:
   - Haemorrhage around the insertion site.
   - Infection around the puncture site which may cause septicaemia.
   - Catheter movement (generally outward) which may result in accidental removal, or ineffective and potentially dangerous infusion of drugs and fluids.
   - Infection caused by inadequate care of the central venous line circuit (see Figure 20.2).

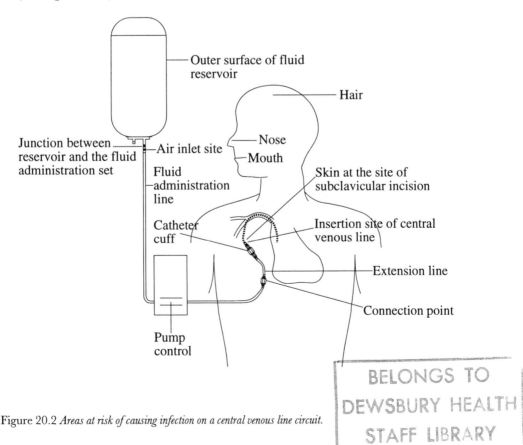

Figure 20.2 *Areas at risk of causing infection on a central venous line circuit.*

Insertion sites

1. Subclavian vein.
2. Internal jugular vein.
3. External jugular vein.
4. Ante-cubital fossa.
5. Femoral vein.

Types of catheter

1. Single lumen, e.g. for parenteral nutrition.
2. Multi-lumen, e.g. for multiple infusions of fluids and drugs.
3. Long lines, e.g. where access to great veins is limited, especially in the burns patient.

1. Procedure for central venous catheterisation

Central venous catheterisation is performed only by a member of the medical staff.

See Chapter 14 on advice on monitoring vital signs and sections 1–5 in chapter 1 for advice on procedures and sharps policy.

Equipment

Sterile intravenous cut down pack
Central venous catheter
Sterile towel
Sterile gown
1 pair of sterile gloves
10 ml syringe
Selection of needles
Skin anaesthetic
Skin antiseptic solution — 10% Povidone Iodine with alcohol or Chlorhexidine
    0.5% (red) with alcohol
20 ml 0.9% saline
Sterile semi-permeable film dressing
Intravenous administration set with attached manometer primed with 0.9% saline
Hand-held suture
Sharps box

Action	Rationale
Observe and record the patient's vital signs.	To detect any changes in the patient's condition.
For subclavian or jugular vein cannulation, position the patient supine with the head tilted downwards. (Trendelenburg position) and with the face turned away from the puncture site.	To reduce the likelihood of air embolism. To engorge central veins and to facilitate their location and puncture (Grant and Todd, 1987).

Action	Rationale
N.B. The Trendelenburg tilt is required only during venous puncture — skin preparation, suturing, etc. The procedure may be performed with the patient lying flat as the head down position may be contra indicated in some patients, e.g. those who are hypertensive.	
The doctor:	
– Examines the potential insertion site.	To locate a suitable insertion site.
– Cleans the skin with the antiseptic solution of choice.	To reduce the risk of infection from the patient's skin flora (Speechly, 1986).
– Infiltrates local anaesthetic into the skin.	To minimise pain and discomfort during the procedure (Sprung and Grenvik, 1985).
– Inserts the cannula (usually using a Seldinger technique).	To assist with insertion of the cannula (Rainbow, 1989).
– Flushes the cannula with saline.	To confirm the patency of the cannula.
– Connects the administration set and manometer to the cannula.	To allow fluid administration and pressure measurement.
– Requests the infusion fluid to be lowered below the level of the patient's heart.	Back flow of venous blood into the administration set confirms that the cannula is positioned in the venous circulation.
– Sutures the cannula to the skin and applies the sterile semi-permeable film dressing in position.	To secure the cannula. To protect the wound from contamination and to allow easy inspection of the site. (Mughal and Leinhardt, 1990).
Reposition the patient appropriately.	To maintain patient safety and comfort.
Record respiratory and cardiovascular observations.	To assess haemodynamic status.
Observe the patient for complications.	To maintain patient safety.
Request a chest X-ray is taken prior to infusion of drugs or fluids.	To confirm the position of the cannula and to exclude pneumothorax (Grant and Todd, 1987).
Record in the appropriate nursing documentation.	To maintain an accurate record.

2. Procedure for recording central venous pressure with a saline manometer

The central venous catheter is connected to an intravenous fluid administration set, a manometer and an extension tube all primed with 0.9% saline. See section 1 in Chapter 1 for advice on procedures.

Action	Rationale
Position the patient flat and supine. If the patient is unable to tolerate lying flat a measurement may be taken in an upright position. Subsequent measurements should be made with the patient in the same position.	To obtain accurate, consistent recordings (Haynes, 1991).
Check the infusion is running freely.	To ensure the catheter is patent.
Line up zero on the manometer with the mid-axillary point. When the manometer is mounted on a dripstand a spirit level should be used. If using a mobile manometer, the column should be held against the patient's chest.	To establish zero prior to measurement and ensure accuracy of readings (Rainbow, 1989).
Single-lumen catheter: "pause" all pumps and switch off infusions for the minimum time necessary to take the recording.	To avoid inaccuracy caused by pressure from pumps and infusions.
N.B. Where drugs and/or fluids are flowing through a single lumen catheter great care must be taken as discontinuation of infusions or inadvertent delivery of bolus doses of drugs may precipitate respiratory and/or cardiovascular complications.	To maintain respiratory and cardiovascular stability.
Multi-lumen catheter: an identified lumen (usually the largest bore) is used.	To allow fluid and/or drug infusions to continue interrupted.
Turn the tap at the base of the measuring column off to the patient and allow the manometer column to fill with saline for up to 20 cm (no more). Do not allow the cotton filter at the top of the manometer to become wet.	To provide a column of fluid against which pressure may be monitored. The cotton filters in the manometer prevent bacterial contamination, but are inactive if they become wet which occurs if the column fills above 20 cm (Rainbow, 1989).
Turn the tap so the fluid from the source is off and saline from the column can run directly into the patient (see Figure 20.4 a and b). Respiratory oscillations will be present if the catheter is correctly positioned.	To allow the fluid level in the column to fall.

Action	Rationale
When the fluid level stops falling, read the lower pressure (i.e. on expiration, in cm of water).	To measure central venous pressure.
Turn the tap to reconnect the infusion to the patient and set the infusion at the prescribed rate.	To re-establish infusions of drugs and/or fluids. To maintain patency of the CVP cannula.
Reposition the patient appropriately.	To maintain patient safety and comfort.
Take CVP readings hourly or as prescribed by the medical staff.	Several recordings show trends which will permit early diagnosis and treatment of hypovolaemia or circulation overload. Normal values lie between 3–15 cm H_2O (Low, 1990).
Record measurement, noting any trends in the recordings and report any changes to the senior nurse.	To monitor the patient's haemodynamic status and to maintain an accurate record.

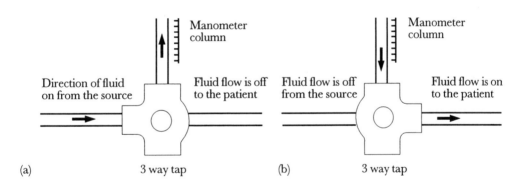

Figure 20.3 *(a) Position for filling the manometer. (b) Position for reading the CVP.*

References

Grant T, Todd E (1987) Enteral and Parenteral Nutrition. 2nd Edition. Oxford: Blackwell Scientific Publications.

Haynes S (1991) Central venous pressure monitoring. Professional Nurse 6 (12): 727–9.

Low JM (1990) Haemodynamic monitoring. In Oh TE, (Ed) Intensive Care Manual 3rd edition. Sydney: Butterworths.

Mughal M, Leinhardt A (1990) Infected feeding lines. Care of the Critically Ill 6: 228–32.

Rainbow C (1989) Monitoring the Critically Ill. London: Heinemann Nursing.

Speechly V (1986) Intravenous therapy: Peripheral central lines. Nursing 3rd Series. The Add-on Journal of Clinical Nursing 3: 95–100.

Sprung CL, Grenvik A (1985) Invasive Procedures in Critical Care. Edinburgh: Churchill Livingstone.

Further Reading

Hollingsworth S (1987) Getting on line. Nursing Times 83 (29): 61–2.

Strong A (1983) Monitoring central venous pressure. Nursing 10: 8–10.

Chapter 21
Care of a patient receiving enteral nutrition

A catabolic burns patient will require dietary assistance to reach the correct calorific and protein intake during the healing phase following burn trauma.

It has been shown that the gastrointestinal tract is the preferred route for supplementation of oral intake in patients following burn injuries. In addition to being considered safer, more economical and more efficient in the utilisation of nutrients than parenteral nutrition, external feeding will preserve gastrointestinal function and mucosal integrity and reduce the incidence of hepatic steatosis and bacterial translocation (Herndon et al., 1987, 1989; Saito et al., 1987).

Indications

All patients with major burn trauma will require adequate nutrition. Enteral feeding should be used in preference to total parenteral nutrition (TPN) in order to reduce the incidence of complications and the risk of gastrointestinal problems (Gregg and Rees, 1970) (see guidelines on parenteral nutrition in Chapter 22).

Enteral nutritional support has been advocated for burn patients to prevent metabolic complications resulting from nutritional deficit, promote wound healing and reduce post burn hypermetabolic responses (Jenkins et al., 1989; Trocki et al., 1995).

Complications

1. Metabolic disturbances.
2. Dehydration.
3. Constipation.
4. Vomiting.
5. Diarrhoea.
6. Abdominal distension.
7. Aspiration pneumonia.
8. Blocked tube.
9. Non-absorption of feed.
10. Reduced appetite.
11. Paralytic ileus.

1. Procedure for passing a nasogastric tube (ryles or fine bore)

Inserting a nasogastric tube involves passing a flexible hollow tube into the stomach or duodenum via the nasopharynx. The fine bore tube should be passed by a member of the medical team or by a registered nurse who is recognised as being competent to perform the procedure. It is the doctor's responsibility however, to ascertain that the tube is in the correct position before feeding commences.

Nasogastric tubes are manufactured from plastic, silicone or PVC in a variety of diameters and lengths (Taylor, 1988). Each patient should be assessed on an individual basis to determine the size and type to be used.

Indications for use

1. Aspirating gastric contents in cases of gastrointestinal obstruction causing paralytic ileus during the initial fluid resuscitation phase following burn trauma (Ryles tube) (Price, 1989).
2. To ensure correct fluid resuscitation when using oral solutions in children who will not tolerate them orally (fine bore tube).
3. Administration of medication to both adults and children if unable to tolerate orally (fine bore tube).
4. Administration of enteral feeding to both adults and children (fine bore tube)

See sections 1, 2 and 5 in Chapter 1 for advice on procedures.

Equipment

Tray/trolley
Nasogastric tube (of appropriate size)
Bowl of cold water to moisten tube
Spigot
Hypo-allergenic tape to secure tube in position
Measuring jug (optional)
20 ml syringe and tube adapter
Blue litmus paper
Gallipot
50 ml syringe
Stethoscope
Water-repellent sheet
Box of tissues
Glass of water if patient conscious and allowed oral fluids
1 pair of unsterile gloves
Jug of water and beaker
Cotton buds (if required)

Action	Rationale
Check by asking the patient or referring to the notes whether or not the patient has had an injury to the nose or undergone nasal surgery. If one nostril has been so affected, use the other one.	Any previous injury may hinder or prevent passage of the tube or cause further injury.
Check the nostrils are clean. Request patient to blow nose as necessary.	Mucus from the nostrils may build up and cause oedema of the nasal mucosa.
Ask the patient to place a finger over each nostril in turn and sniff with the other nostril.	To check the nostril selected is patent.
Check the length of the tube to be passed by measuring the distance from the base of the sternum to mouth to the tip of the ear lobe. Note the marking on the tube.	To ensure the tube is the correct length to enter the stomach (Delaney, 1991).
If the patient is conscious arrange a signal by which the patient can request the nurse to halt the procedure.	The patient will then feel in control.
Sit the patient in an upright position (unless contraindicated) and ensure the head is well supported by pillows.	The patient's natural reaction is to move the head backwards as the nurse starts to pass the tube.
Apply the water repellent sheet around the neck and over the chest.	To prevent wetting and/or soiling of bed linen.
Ask the patient to bend the head slightly forward.	This will close the glottis and prevent the tube entering the bronchus (Methaney, 1988).
Apply the unsterile gloves.	To protect the nurse from body fluids.
Dip the end of the tube into cold water.	To facilitate passage of the tube.
Pass the end of the tube into the selected nostril in an upwards and backwards direction. If an obstruction is felt, withdraw the tube, wipe it and try again in a slightly different direction or use the other nostril.	In order to follow the natural line of the nasal pathway (Delaney, 1991).
The passage of the tube may be advanced by asking the patient to swallow repeatedly — sips of water can be taken to aid this.	To ensure the tube is advanced into the stomach.
Advance the tube at a speed acceptable to the patient to the appropriate marking ensuring it is not coiled at the back of the mouth/throat.	To ensure patient's co-operation. To ensure the tube is advanced into the stomach.
Secure the tube with hypo-allergenic tape to the nose.	To prevent dislodging of the tube once in position (Price, 1989).

Action	Rationale
N.B. If a fine bore tube is used remove the wire (never reintroduce the wire when the tube is _in situ_).	Reintroducing the wire may perforate the tube and the gastrointestinal tract (Crocker, Krey and Steffee, 1981).
Check the position of the tube.	
– Using the 20 ml syringe, aspirate a few millilitres of gastric content, release into the gallipot and test with blue litmus paper.	Acid gastric content will turn blue litmus red and confirm the tube is in the stomach (Methaney et al., 1989).
– Place a stethoscope over the epigastric region. Using a 50 ml syringe inject 5–10 ml air in one movement into the tube and asculate over the epigastric region (a "whoosh" sound will be heard).	It is possible to rupture fine bore tubes by using excessive force with a small syringe (Anderton et al, 1986). A whoosh sound will indicate the end of the tube is in the stomach.
Measure total aspirate if using a Ryles tube (if required), and note colour/odour and any abnormalities.	To aid diagnosis (Methaney, 1988; Methaney et al., 1989).
Close the tube with the attached bung or spigot.	To prevent leakage.
Remove gloves and wash hands.	
Record the results of the procedure in the appropriate nursing documentation.	To maintain an accurate record.
N.B. Frequent mouth care will be necessary if the patient is ordered nil by mouth.	

2. Procedure for administering nasogastric feed via a fine bore tube

Feeding regimes are planned with the assistance of the dietician. See sections 1, 2 and 5 in Chapter 1 for advice on procedures.

Equipment

Enteral feed regime
Prescribed feed (commercially prepared in a glass bottle or enteral feeding solution and reservoir bag)
Dripstand
Feed administration set
Feed pump
Jug
20 ml syringe

Jug of water
Additive label
Label for administration set
Fluid balance chart

Action	Rationale
Prepare prescribed feed and check the expiry date.	To ensure correct feed is administered and that it is not out of date.
Attach the completed additive label to the bottle/reservoir.	To maintain an accurate record of the bottle/reservoir contents.
Prime the feed administration set.	To remove air from the line, thus reducing the risk of gastric distension.
Check the position of the tube:	
− Test the aspirate with blue litmus paper.	Acid gastric content will turn blue litmus red and confirm the tube is in the stomach (Methaney et al., 1989).
− Inject 20 ml of air into the stomach and listen for its entry.	To ascertain the position of the tube in the stomach (Miller, Tomlinson and Sahn, 1985).
− Request a chest X-ray.	To ascertain the position of the tube (Henley, 1989; Delaney, 1991).
N.B. Do not commence feed if there is any doubt about the correct position of the tube.	
Flush the tube with 30 ml of water. (Sterile water should only be used if the patient is immunocompromised.)	To maintain patency of the tube (Taylor and Goodinson-McLaren, 1992).
Attach the administration set to the nasogastric tube.	To allow the feed to commence.
Commence the feed at the prescribed rate.	To ensure delivery of the feed at the prescribed rate.
Label the administration set and reservoir.	To maintain an accurate record.
Record in the appropriate nursing documentation and on a fluid balance chart.	To maintain an accurate record and to assist in the detection of dehydration/fluid overload.
Change the administration set and reservoir every 24 hours.	To minimise the risk of infection.

3. Procedure for care of a patient receiving nasogastric feeding via a fine bore tube

Enteral nutrition is administered via a fine bore nasogastric tube, an administration set attached to a reservoir, or feeding bag and connected to a feed pump.

Action	Rationale
Store the feed at room temperature prior to administration.	Feeds straight from the fridge may cause diarrhoea (Gormicon, 1970), and those too warm are at risk of contamination from harmful pathogens.
Ensure the patient is receiving the prescribed volume of the correct feed and chart the amount.	To ensure delivery of the correct type and volume of feed as requested by the dietician.
Flush the nasogastric tube with 30 ml of water after each bottle or bag of feed.	To prevent blockage of the tube.
N.B. A 50 ml syringe should be used for administration of medication via the tube and for flushing the tube.	A smaller bore syringe will increase the tube space pressure and there is a danger of the tube rupturing under the pressure (Taylor, 1988).
Change the giving set every 24 hours, and discard any remaining feed.	To prevent infection and/or stomach irritation
Monitor bowel function daily.	To enable bowel complications to be detected and treated early.
Check the patient's blood sugar levels as directed by the medical staff.	To detect signs of hypo or hyperglycaemia.
Monitor and assess the patient's nutritional status as appropriate using:	To ensure adequate nutrition requirements are maintained (Henley, 1989).
– Serum urea and electrolyte measurements (twice weekly).	To assess catabolic status.
– Urine urea and electrolyte measurements (24 hour collections, twice weekly)	
– Weight of the patient (with dressings, twice weekly).	Twice weekly weight will assess if nutritional requirements are being met (Bell and Wyatt, 1986).
Record any results in the appropriate nursing documentation.	To maintain an accurate record.

References

Anderton A et al. (1986) Microbiological control in enteral feeding. A Guidance Document Prepared for the Committee of the Pen Group. London: British Diabetic Association.

Bell SJ, Wyatt J (1986) Nutrition guidelines for burned patients. Journal of American Dietetic Association 86: 648.

Crocker K, Krey S, Steffee W (1981) Performance evaluation of a new naso-gastric feeding tube. Journal of Parenteral and Enteral Nutrition 1: 80–2.

Delaney C (1991) Naso-gastric intubation use and abuse. Surgical Nurse 4 (3) 4–9.

Gormicon A (1970) Pre-packaged tube feeding. Hospital 144: 58–60.

Gregg SH, Rees OM (1970) Scientific Principles of Nursing. St. Louis: CV Mosby.

Henley M (1989) Feed that burn. Journal of the International Society for Burn Injuries 15 (6) 351–61.

Herndon DN, Barrow RE, Stein MD et al. (1989) Increased mortality with intravenous supplemental feeding in severely burned patients. Journal of Burn Care and Rehabilitation 10: 309.

Herndon DN, Stein MD, Rutan TC et al. (1987) Failure of TPN supplementation to improve liver function immunity and mortality in thermally injured patients. Journal of Trauma 27: 195.

Jenkins M, Gottschlich MM, Alexander JW et al. (1989) Enteral alimentation in the early post burn phase. Cited in Blackburn GL, Bell SJ, Mullen JL (Eds) Nutritional Medicine. A Case Management Approach. Philadelphia: WB Saunders. p 1.

Methaney N (1988) Measures to test placement of naso-gastric and naso-intestinal feeding tubes: a review. Nursing Research 37 (6): 324–9.

Methaney N, Williams P et al. (1989) Effectiveness of pH measurements in predicting feeding tube placement. Nursing Research 38 (5) 280–5.

Miller KS, Tomlinson JR, Sahn SA (1985) Pleuropulmonary complications of enteral tube feeding. 88: 230–3.

Price B (1989) Naso-gastric intubation. Nursing Times 85 (13) 50–2.

Saito H, Trocki O, Alexander JW et al. (1987) The route of nutrient administration on the nutritional state, catabolic hormone secretion and gut mucosal integrity after burn injury. Journal of parenteral and enteral nutrition 11: 1.

Taylor S, Goodinson-McLaren SM (1992) Nutritional Support — A Team Approach. London: Wolfe Publishing.

Taylor SJ (1988) A guide to naso-gastric feeding. Professional Nurse 3 (11): 439–42.

Trocki O, Michelini JA, Robbins ST, Eichelberger MR (1995) Evaluation of early enteral feeding children less than 3 years old with smaller burns (8–25 percent TBSA). Journal of the International Society for Burn Injuries 21 (1): 17.

Further Reading

Grant T, Todd E (1987) Enteral and Parenteral Nutrition. Oxford: Blackwell Scientific Publications.

Jones E (1982) Nursing aspects of tube feeding. Nursing 12 (4): 34–47.

Sutherland AB (1985) Nutrition and general factors influencing infection in burns. Journal of Hospital Infection 6 (3): 31–42.

Chapter 22
Care of a patient receiving parenteral nutrition

Parenteral nutrition is the intravenous administration of a balanced diet in elemental form. Carbohydrate is usually administered in the form of dextrose, fat as soya emulsion, and protein as amino acids. Trace elements, vitamins and electrolyte solutions are included in the regime.

Indications

Intravenous feeding is more hazardous and more expensive than enteral feeding and is only employed when the gut is non-functional or when it is unable to cope with the load necessary to maintain nutritional balance (Sutherland, 1985). When total parenteral nutrition (TPN) is administered the patient's intake is matched as closely as possible with his or her requirements.

The feeding system

The feeding system comprises a bag of nutrients, an intravenous administration set with an additional extension tube and a central venous cannula. The aim of care is to maintain sterility of the system as a whole. It is a closed circuit which is broken only once daily when a new infusion of nutrients is commenced. The system is used exclusively for TPN, no ramps or taps are added to the infusion lines and no additional fluids or drugs are given via the system.

Sites

The subclavian veins are normally used because TPN cannulae are subcutaneously tunnelled. Internal jugular veins may be used but tunnelling is more difficult here.

Complications

It is the nurse's role to be aware of complications that may develop and to be aware of observations that should be undertaken routinely (Atkins, 1989).

1. Infection. TPN lines may be a focus for infection. If no other cause for a pyrexia can be found in a febrile patient the TPN cannula is usually removed.
2. Air embolus.

3. Leaks and disconnection.
4. Blocked cannula.
5. Great vein thrombosis. Unilateral, warm swelling of the arm on the side of the feeding line indicates venous thrombosis.
6. Metabolic disturbances, e.g. hyperglycaemia.
7. Rebound hypoglycaemia when the feed is discontinued.
8. Subcutaneous extroversion or pleural effusion.
9. All the potential complications of central venous catheterisation.

Monitoring (Henley, 1989)

Routine burn care observations should be recorded. Particular attention should be paid to fluid balance and signs of infection. In addition:

1. Daily blood specimens:
   - for urea, creatinine, electrolytes, osmolality and glucose, in addition to 4–6 hourly Reflocheck measurements (Hopkinson and Davies, 1987).
   - for full blood count and platelets.
2. Twice weekly 24-hour urine collection for urea, creatinine, electrolytes and osmolality.
3. Daily urinalysis.
4. Twice weekly blood specimens:
   - for liver function tests.
   - for calcium, magnesium, phosphate and zinc levels.
5. Weekly blood specimens:
   - for clotting screen.

1. Procedure for insertion of a TPN catheter

This procedure is carried out by the medical staff assisted by a nurse. TPN catheters are tunnelled subcutaneously to minimise the risks of infection and to stabilise the catheter for long-term use. Full aseptic techniques must be undertaken.

See sections 1–5 in Chapter 1 for advice on procedures and sharps policy.

Equipment

Trolley
Water repellent sheet
Sterile intravenous cut-down pack
Sterile gown and towel pack
Sterile linen sheets
1 pair of sterile gloves
3 x 10 ml syringes
Selection of needles
Local anaesthetic agent

Ampoules of heparinised saline

Skin antiseptic — 10% Povidone Iodine with alcohol or Chlorhexidine 0.5% (red) with alcohol

2 sterile semi-permeable film dressings (of choice)

Central venous catheter (of choice)

No. 11 sterile blade

Suture 2/0 silk

Sharps box

Volumetric pump and appropriate giving set

500 ml bag of 0.9% saline

Extension set and closed intravenous connection system (click lock)

Action	Rationale
Remove the bed head and protect the bed linen, using water repellent sheets.	To prepare the environment for the procedure.
Lay the patient flat on the bed, one pillow may be placed longitudinally under the shoulder blades.	Raising the clavicle allows easier venepuncture.
At the request of the doctor raise the foot of the bed (Trendelenburg position).	Position increases venous filling and reduces risk of air embolism.
Ask the patient to turn his or her head away from the insertion site.	Facilitates easy access (Grant and Todd, 1987).
Observe and record the patient's vital signs.	To detect any changes in the patient's condition.
The nurse:	
— Opens the intravenous cut-down set onto the trolley.	To maintain a sterile technique.
— Opens the gown and towel set and the gloves for the doctor.	
The doctor puts on the gown and gloves and opens out the i.v. cut-down set onto the trolley.	To maintain a sterile technique.
The nurse:	
— Opens the supplementary items onto the sterile field.	
— Checks the antiseptic solution of choice with the doctor and pours into the gallipot.	Reduces the risk of errors in administration.

Action	Rationale
− Checks the local anaesthetic and heparinised saline with the doctor.	
The doctor:	
− Examines the potential insertion site.	To locate insertion site.
− Cleans the skin with the antiseptic solution of choice and allows to air dry.	To minimise the risk of infection.
− Infiltrates the local anaesthetic into the skin.	To minimise pain and discomfort during the procedure.
− Inserts the catheter.	
− Flushes the catheter with the heparinised saline.	To confirm patency of catheter.
− Connects the primed extension set, closed i.v. connection system and administration set to the catheter.	Allows administration of fluid.
− Sutures the catheter to the skin.	To secure the catheter.
− Applies sterile semi-permeable film dressings to the insertion and exit sites.	To minimise the risk of cross infection and facilitate easy inspection of the sites.
Reposition the patient comfortably and record vital signs.	To maintain comfort of the patient and to detect any changes in the patient's condition.
The doctor will arrange a chest X-ray to be performed.	To confirm the position of the catheter (Grant and Todd, 1987).
The doctor will confirm the correct position of the catheter and record it in the patient's case notes prior to commencing the TPN feed.	Reduces errors in administration of TPN feed.
The nurse will record the procedure in the appropriate documentation.	To maintain an accurate record.

2. Procedure for changing a TPN bag

The TPN bag is changed at approximately 1800 hours daily and residual feed is discarded. Administration sets must be changed every 72 hours and the click-lock housing must be changed every time the administration set is changed.

See sections 1,2 and 5 in Chapter 1 for advice on procedures.

Equipment

Trolley
Alcohol hand rub solution
Alcohol based wipe x 2

TPN bag cover
TPN bag
Patient's prescription chart

Action	Rationale
Check the TPN bag (contents, batch number, patient's name and expiry date) against the prescription card with a second nurse.	To ensure that the patient receives the correct feed and it is not out of date.
Place light protective cover over TPN bag if it contains water-soluble vitamins.	Protecting the solution from light prevents the vitamin content of TPN fluid being destroyed (Grant and Todd, 1987).
Fold back the cover to expose the port and lay the bag on one side of the trolley.	Provides easy access.
Close the roll clamp on the administration set.	Temporarily turns off the infusion.
Place the current TPN bag next to the new bag on the trolley.	To maintain easy access.
Clean hands with alcohol hand rub solution.	To minimise the risk of cross infection.
Open one alcohol wipe, swab port and lid on new TPN bag and allow to air dry.	To minimise the risk of cross infection — alcohol destroys most micro-organisms.
Open second alcohol wipe, swab port and top section of the administration set chamber and allow to air dry.	To minimise the risk of infection as bacteria agglutinate and die (Lee and Vankat Raman, 1990).
Tear lid from port without touching the newly exposed end of the port.	To prevent contamination of spike which could contaminate TPN fluid.
Hang up new TPN bag.	
Check there are no air bubbles in the administration set.	To commence the new infusion.
Open the roll clamp.	To facilitate flow.
Commence the infusion at the prescribed rate.	To ensure the feed is delivered at the prescribed rate.
Record in the appropriate documentation.	To maintain an accurate record.

3. Procedure for changing the TPN bag and administration set

Administration sets and the click-lock housing connections must be changed every 72 hours. The TPN feed is changed every 24 hours.

See sections 1–5 in Chapter 1 for advice on procedures.

Equipment

Trolley
Alcohol hand rub solution
2 alcohol-based wipes
TPN feed
Protective bag cover
Administration set
Closed i.v. connection system (click-lock)
Patient's prescription chart
Disposal bag

Action	Rationale
Check the TPN bag (contents, batch number, patient's name, and expiry date) against the prescription card with a second nurse.	To ensure the patient receives the correct feed and it is not out of date, to minimise errors in administration of feed.
Place light protective cover over TPN bag.	Protecting the solution from light prevents the vitamin content of TPN being destroyed (Grant and Todd, 1987)
Hang the new TPN bag from the dripstand.	
Fold back cover to expose port.	Provides easy access.
Remove administration set from sterile packaging and close roller clamp.	To prepare administration set for use.
Clean hands with alcohol hand rub solution.	To minimise the risk of cross infection.
Open alcohol wipe, swab port and lid on TPN bag and allow to air dry.	To minimise infection. Alcohol destroys most micro-organisms.
Remove protective cover from spike of administration set and insert into port of TPN bag.	To connect new administration set to TPN feed bag.
Open the roller clamp and prime the administration set with feed. Check there are no air bubbles in the tubing. Close the roller clamp.	To remove air from the administration set tubing and prevent air embolism.
Remove closed i.v. connection system from sterile packaging and attach to free end of administration set. Prime with feed.	To complete new TPN circuit.
Close roller clamp on existing TPN feed administration set. Switch volumetric pump off and remove tubing from machine.	To cease flow of TPN feed and to allow insertion of new TPN circuit into volumetric pump.
Insert new administration set into the volumetric pump, switch on machine and set it to "hold".	To prepare volumetric pump for use.

Action	Rationale
Clamp extension line attached to TPN catheter.	To minimise the risk of infection and prevent air embolism or leakage of blood.
Disconnect existing closed i.v. connection system and old administration set from extension line and place in disposal bag.	To allow new circuit to be connected.
Clean hands with alcohol hand rub solution.	To minimise the risk of infection.
Using second alcohol wipe, swab extension line port and allow to air dry.	To minimise the risk of cross infection. Alcohol destroys most micro-organisms (Lee and Vankat Raman, 1990).
Remove protective cover from closed i.v. connection system and connect to extension line.	To complete the TPN circuit.
Unclamp extension line.	To facilitate flow.
Open roller clamp and turn on volumetric pump.	To facilitate flow.
Commence infusion at prescribed rate.	To ensure feed is delivered at the prescribed rate.
Record in the appropriate documentation.	To maintain an accurate record.

4. Procedure for redressing the TPN catheter site

The dressing should remain intact at all times and should be replaced every 7 days unless it becomes loose in the meantime.

See sections 1–5 in Chapter 1 for advice on procedures.

Equipment

Trolley
Sterile dressing pack
1 pair of unsterile gloves
1 pair of sterile gloves
Skin antiseptic solution — 10% Povidone Iodine with alcohol, Chlorhexidine
        0.5% (red) with alcohol
Sterile towel
Bacteriological wound swab
Semi-permeable film dressings (of choice)
Disposal bag

Action	Rationale
Apply the unsterile gloves and remove dressings from the catheter insertion site and the exit site.	To expose the catheter sites and allow for observation and wound cleaning.
Discard into the disposal bag.	To minimise the risk of infection.
Remove gloves and wash hands.	To minimise the risk of infection.
Apply sterile gloves, open pack and place sterile towel around the catheter site.	To maintain asepsis.
If the insertion or exit site appears red, inflamed, smells or is oozing purulent discharge take a bacteriological wound swab for culture and sensitivity label and send to the microbiology laboratory.	To isolate any micro-organisms that may cause infections (Mughal and Leinhardt, 1990)
Clean the insertion and exit sites individually with the skin antiseptic solution of choice.	To remove any blood or other exudate which may encourage the growth of micro-organisms.
Apply the sterile semi-permeable film dressing of choice to the insertion and exit sites.	To secure the catheter in position. To protect the insertion and exit sites from contamination and to allow easy viewing of the sites (Mughal and Leinhardt, 1990).
Apply an elastic supportive dressing to the catheter away from the insertion site.	To avoid traction and or drag on the line and possible catheter removal (Lee and Vankat Raman, 1990).
Ensure TPN feed is infused at the prescribed rate.	To ensure feed is delivered at prescribed rate.
Record in the appropriate documentation.	To maintain an accurate record.

References

Atkins S (1989) Parenteral nutrition — The nurse's role. Surgical Nurse. Feb: 31.
Grant T, Todd E (1987) Enteral and Parenteral Nutrition. Oxford: Blackwell Scientific Publications.
Henley M (1989) Feed that burn. Burns Journal 15 (6) 351–61.
Hopkinson RB, Davies B (1987) A guide to parenteral feeding. Care of the Critically Ill. 3 (3): 16–18.
Lee HA, Vankat Raman G (1990) A Handbook of Parenteral Nutrition. London: Chapman and Hall.
Mughal M, Leinhardt A (1990) Infection feeding lines. Care of the Critically Ill. 6 (6): 29.
Sutherland AB (1985) Nutrition and general factors influencing infection in burns. Journal of Hospital Infection 6 (B): 31–42.

Further Reading

Banergee A (1988) Total Parenteral Nutrition in the Intensive Care Unit. Care of the Critically Ill 4 (5) 8–11.
Childs C, Hall T, Davenport PJ, Little RA (1990) Dietary intake and changes in body weight in burned children. Burns Journal 16 (6): 418–22.
Chuang J, Chuang S (1991) Implications of a distant septic focus in parenteral nutrition catheter colonisation. Journal of Parenteral and Enteral Nutrition 15: 173–5.
Conley JM, Grieves K, Peters B (1989) A prospective, randomised study comparing transparent and dry gauze dressings for central venous catheters. Journal of Infectious Disease 159: 310–19.

Elliott TSJ (1993) Line associated bacteraemias. Communicable Diseases Report 3: 91–6.

Gibilso PA et al. (1986) *In vitro* contamination of "piggyback"/"heparin lock" assemblies: Prevention of contamination with a closed, positive locking device (click-lock) Journal of Parenteral and Enteral Nutrition 10: 431–3.

Goodinson SM (1990) Keeping the flora out. Recurring the risk of infection in i.v. therapy. Professional Nurse August: 572–5.

Grimble GK (1989) TPN novel energy substrates. Intensive Therapy and Clinical Monitoring 10 (4): 108–13.

Holmes S (1987) Nutrition in the critically ill. Care of the Critically Ill. 15: 17.

Maki DG (1991) Prospective randomised trial of povidone iodine, alcohol and chlorhexidine for the prevention of infection associated with central venous and arterial catheters. Lancet 338: 339–43.

Yoshifumi I et al. (1992) Experimental study of hub contamination: Effect of a new connection device: The I system. Journal of Parenteral and Enteral Nutrition 16: 178–80.

Chapter 23
Care of a patient receiving epidural analgesia

Epidural analgesia is achieved by infusing local anaesthetic or analgesic solution into the epidural space through a fine bore tube indwelling catheter, either intermittently or by a continuous infusion (see Figure 23.1).

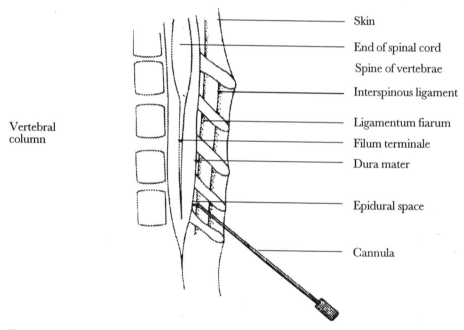

Figure 23.1 *Cross section of the veterbral column illustrating entry of epidural cannula.*
(From Mallett and Bailey: Royal Marsden NHS Trust Manual of Clinical Nursing Procedures 4th Ed (1996) reproduced with permission of Blackwell Science, Oxford)

This technique provides analgesia, reflex muscle flaccidity, a degree of hypotension and ischaemia secondary to sympathetic blockage while allowing spontaneous respiration to continue relatively unimpaired (Pritchard and David, 1989).

The epidural space

The epidural space lies within the vertebral column between the dura mater and the walls of the vertebral canal. All the nerves leaving the spinal cord pass through it, surrounded by their coverings or dura.

198

Anterior and posterior nerve roots of all spinal nerves traverse the epidural space, therefore injection of a local analgesic or anaesthetic solution into the space where nerves carrying pain sensations from the site of injury enter through the intervertebral foramina to join the spinal cord produces an epidural block (see Figure 23.2).

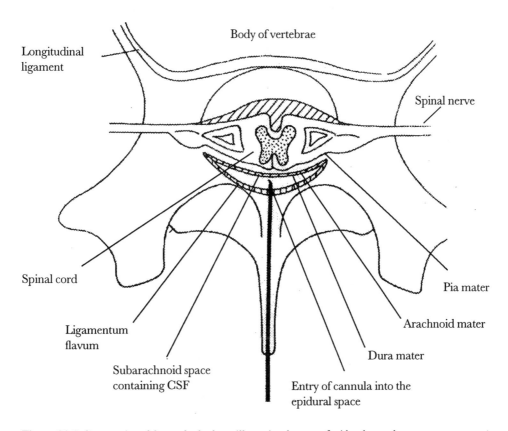

Figure 23.2 *Cross-section of the vertebral column illustrating the entry of epidural cannula.*

The motor and sensory fibres vary in size and susceptibility to different strengths of analgesia and anaesthetic solution. Thus selective nerve block can be performed where afferent pain sensation only is prevented, whilst efferent motor impulses are unimpaired.

Several factors affect the choice of drug used. Narcotic analgesics given epidurally inhibit transmission of pain sensation to the higher brain centres. Thus, drugs administered via this route must be free of potentially neurotoxic substances such as preservatives and additives (Haight, 1987).

Epidural drugs

Epidural "top ups", i.e. the administration of a bolus dose of drug via the epidural cannula are performed only by anaesthetists or qualified members of the medical staff. Continuous epidural infusion may be administered only by nurses who have been specially trained to perform the procedure.

Drugs currently used include:

1. Bupivacaine 0.125–0.75% solution, which resembles lignocaine but is slightly less toxic, although considered more potent. Its effect is variable but it may provide analgesia for up to 8 hours (Pritchard and David, 1989).
2. Morphine 2–4 mg in 5–10 ml 0.9% saline may provide analgesia for up to 10 hours (Pritchard and David, 1989).
3. Diamorphine 5 mg.

Opioid receptors in the brain and spinal cord have been discovered, leading to the use of epidural opioids. Potential advantages are pain relief without complications of motor block, sympathetic block or numbness. Some respiratory depression may occur. Opioids may be added to epidural infusions of bupivacaine to enhance analgesia.

Factors affecting the spread of solution in the epidural space include:

1. Volume. Spread occurs up and down the space from the site of injection, and the degree of spread depends on the volume of solution being delivered.
2. Gravity.
3. Site of injection. Analgesia is centred on the site of injection occurring in a segmental band.
4. Rate of injection. Rapid injection increases the degree of spread.
5. Concentration. A given volume of a more concentrated solution spreads further than the same volume of a lower concentration using the same drug.

Indications for epidural analgesia in the Burns Unit

In many cases epidural analgesia is used to provide localised pain relief without the respiratory depression associated with systemic analgesia, e.g. intravenous or intramuscular opioids. Patients who benefit from epidural analgesia include those who have undergone surgery to lower extremities, e.g. to reduce pain in donor areas and skin grafted areas.

Absolute contraindications

1. Pre-existing infection at the puncture site.
2. A patient on a full anticoagulation regime or whose clotting is severely deranged due to disease. Rupture of blood vessels in the epidural space during cannulation could cause epidural haematoma.

Complications of epidural analgesia (Pritchard and David, 1989)

1. Sympathetic nerve fibres arise from the spinal cord between the first thoracic and third lumbar segments. Blockage results in reduced peripheral resistance, vasodilation, hypotension, venous pooling, falling cardiac output and further hypotension.

Hypotension following epidural "top up" occurs suddenly and must be corrected immediately by rapid infusion of intravenous fluid. Ephedrine may be required to restore blood pressure.

2. Tenderness over the puncture site.
3. Haematoma due to bleeding into the epidural space.
4. Infection.
5. Toxic effects due to overdose.
6. Breakage of the catheter within the epidural space.
7. Accidental catheter removal.
8. Persistent slight motor or sensory weakness.
9. Because the epidural space is only a few millimetres across it is easy to advance the needle in too far, accidentally puncturing the dura mater. Local analgesia solution may then reach the brain, affecting the cranial nerves, respiratory and vasomotor centres. Respiratory paralysis, hypertension and coma may result. The patient must be resuscitated and artificially ventilated until the local analgesia loses its effect. Migration of the cannula through the dura mater following uneventful "top up" has been reported, leading to "total spinal block" some hours after the insertion of the cannula.
10. Headache following inadvertent dural puncture.
11. Paraplegia caused by cord infarction or stenosis of the vertebral canal.
12. Intraoccular haemorrhage caused by a rapid injection of fluid raising the pressure of cerebrospinal fluid.
13. Backache from local irritation of the needle or catheter.
14. Extradural abscess.

Adverse reactions (Haight, 1987)

1. Respiratory depression.
2. Urinary retention.
3. Pruritis.
4. Nausea and vomiting.

1. Procedure for epidural cannulation

Epidural cannulation is performed only by an anaesthetist. Facilities for emergency intubation and ventilation must be available in case of accidental respiratory muscle paralysis. An intravenous infusion must be *in situ* to allow rapid infusion of drugs and/or fluid should hypotension occur.

See sections 1–5 in Chapter 1 for advice on procedures and sharps policy.

Equipment

Sterile lumbar puncture pack
Sterile epidural minipack
1 pair of sterile gloves

5 ml syringe
Selection of needles
Number 11 blade
Local anaesthetic agent
Skin antiseptic solution — 10% Povidone Iodine solution with alcohol or
    Chlorhexidine 0.5% (red) with alcohol
Sterile semi-permeable film dressing
Waterproof tape 2.5 cm wide
Epidural analgesia or anaesthetic as prescribed by the anaesthetist
Patient's prescription chart
Sharps box

Action	Rationale
Record the patient's blood pressure	To provide a baseline measurement for assessment of haemodynamic stability (Gardner, 1992).
Position the patient as requested by the anaesthetist. Usual postures are:	To curve the spine and separate the vertebrae facilitating cannulation (Bragg, 1989).
— The lumbar puncture position: the patient lies on his or her side with knees flexed and brought up towards the chest and with the head forward.	To increase the size of the interlaminar spaces, for maximum flexion of the lumbar vertebrae (Haight, 1987).
— Sit the patient on the edge of the bed, feet resting on a foot stool leaning forwards onto pillows stacked on a bed table.	
Expose the patient's back.	To allow access to the area to be cannulated.
The doctor:	
— Cleans the skin with the antiseptic solution of choice.	To maintain asepsis (Bragg, 1989).
— Instils the local anaesthetic into the skin.	To minimise pain and discomfort for the patient during the procedure (Bragg, 1989).
— Inserts the epidural needle between vertebrae L3 and L4.	To locate the epidural space (Haight, 1987).
— Passes a fine bore cannula through the needle and withdraws the needle leaving the cannula in the epidural space.	To provide access for administration of analgesia.
— Gives a "test dose" of analgesia by bolus injection.	To assess the effectiveness of analgesia (Bragg, 1989).
— Connects the infusion to the cannula.	To provide a continuous flow of analgesia.

Action	Rationale
Apply the sterile semi-permeable film dressing over the insertion site.	To protect the wound from contamination. To secure the cannula in position and to allow easy viewing of the insertion site (Keenlyside, 1992).
Apply waterproof tape around the semi-permeable film dressing and secure the cannula to the patient's back taping the administration port over the patient's shoulder.	To secure the cannula in position (Haight, 1987; Bragg, 1989).
Reposition the patient appropriately.	To maintain patient safety and comfort.
Record the patient's blood pressure every 5 minutes for the first 20 minutes following drug administration.	To detect rapid hypotension (Yarde, 1989).
Observe the patient for complications.	To maintain patient safety (Yarde, 1989).
Record in the appropriate documentation.	To maintain an accurate record.

2. Procedure for administering epidural analgesia by continuous infusion

Only nurses with the appropriate training may carry out this procedure. Only anaesthetists may connect extension tubing to the epidural cannula and give "top ups", i.e. bolus injections.

Facilities for emergency intubation and ventilation must be available and an intravenous infusion must be in place.

See sections 1–3 in Chapter 1 for advice on procedures and sharps policy.

Equipment

> Syringe pump
> 50 ml syringe
> Needle
> Drug additive label
> Prescribed drug
> Sharps box
> Patient's prescription chart

Action	Rationale
Two first level nurses prepare the infusion as prescribed on the patient's prescription chart.	To ensure correct preparation of the infusion.
Close the miniclip clamp on the extension tubing, or occlude the tubing with forceps.	To prevent accidental administration of the drug. To prevent leakage from the epidural cannula.

Action	Rationale
Replace the empty syringe with the newly prepared syringe without contaminating the open ends of the tubing or syringe.	To connect new infusion. Reduces the risk of introducing micro-organisms into the catheter.
Secure the new syringe into the syringe pump and clamp into position.	To secure the infusion into the pump.
Release the miniclip clamp or forceps and start the pump at the prescribed infusion rate.	To allow the infusion to commence.
Monitor the patient's pain level.	To assess the effectiveness of the infusion.
Monitor the patient for complications and adverse reactions.	To ensure the patient's safety (Yarde, 1989).
Protect and inspect the integrity of the strapping whenever the patient is moved, or when the syringe is changed.	To prevent displacement of the cannula.
Record on the patient's prescription chart.	To maintain an accurate record.

3. Procedure for the removal of an epidural cannula

Epidural analgesia in most cases brings about almost complete pain relief. Administration of the chosen drug by bolus or continuous infusion is an expanded role for nurses.

See sections 1–5 in Chapter 1 for advice on procedures.

Equipment

Trolley
Sterile dressing pack
Sachet of normal saline and alcohol swab
1 pair of sterile gloves
1 pair of unsterile gloves
Occlusive plastic dressing spray (optional)
Sterile dressing (of choice)
Sterile scissors
Universal specimen pot
Skin antiseptic solution — 10% Povidone Iodine solution with alcohol or Chlorhexidine 0.5% (red) with alcohol
Disposal bag

Action	Rationale
Apply unsterile gloves. Remove the original dressing from the cannula insertion site and discard into the disposal bag.	To minimise the risk of hand contamination with micro-organisms (Wilson, 1992). To allow access to the cannula site.
Remove gloves and wash hands.	To minimise the risk of infection (Wilson, 1992).
Apply sterile gloves and if exudate is present clean the skin around the insertion site with the antiseptic solution of choice.	To minimise the risk of infection spreading upwards along the cannula tract. To facilitate easy removal of the epidural cannula.
Ask the patient to lie on his or her side with the knees drawn upwards towards the chest in a flexed position, or in a sitting position with the back flexed.	To aid the removal of the cannula (Yarde, 1989).
Remove the cannula by applying gentle traction to the cannula close to the point of entry of the skin.	To facilitate easy removal of the cannula (Yarde, 1989).
Following removal of the cannula inspect the tip and depth of marks along the barrel.	To ensure the cannula has been removed, intact and none has broken off (Yarde, 1989).
N.B. If any of the cannula has been left *in situ* apply a sterile dressing and inform the doctor.	
Apply a sterile dressing (of choice) to the puncture site and leave *in situ* for 24 hours.	To minimise the access of micro-organisms along the cannula tract (Sheldon, 1994).
Record in the appropriate nursing documentation.	To maintain an accurate record.

References

Bragg CL (1989) Practical aspects of epidural and intrathecal narcotic analgesia in the intensive care setting. Heart Lung 18 (6): 599–608.

Gardner AM (1992) Epidural analgesia — monitoring aspects. Surgical Nurse 5 (4): 10–13.

Haight K (1987) What you should know about epidural analgesia. Nursing 58–9.

Keenlyside D (1992) Detail counts — infection control in i.v. therapy. Professional Nurse 17 (4) 226–32.

Pritchard AP, David JA (1989) Epidural analgesia. In Pritchard AP, David JA (Eds) Manual of Clinical Nursing Procedures (2nd Edition) London: Harper and Row. pp 150–1.

Sheldon JE (1994) What you should know about i.v. dressings. Nursing 24 (8): 32.

Wilson J (1992) Theory and practice of isolation nursing. Nursing Standard 6 (17): 30–1.

Yarde A (1989) Epidural analgesia. Professional Nurse 4 (12): 608–13.

Further Reading

Bibbings J (1984) Epidural analgesia. Nursing Times 80 (35): 52–5.

Litwack K et al. (1989) Practical points in the management of continuous epidural infusion. Journal of Post Anaesthetic Nursing 4 (5): 327–30.

Sheargold L (1986) Epidural and spinal anaesthetics. Nursing Times 82 (2): 44–5.

Chapter 24
Care of a patient with a split skin graft

A skin graft is a section of epidermis and dermis (Alderman, 1988; Coull, 1991) that has been completely separated from its blood supply and transplanted to another area of the body (see Figure 24.1). It can be applied in sheets, or meshed to cover a larger area.

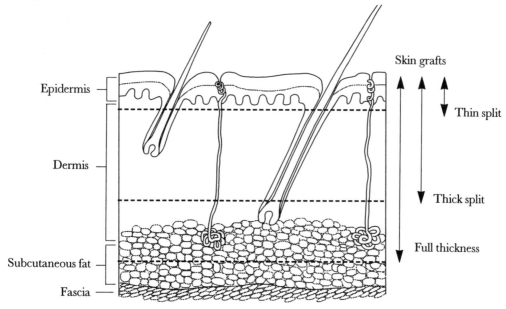

Figure 24.1 *The layers of skin showing depth of skin grafts.*

Partial thickness, split or Thiersch grafts are taken in sheets using a blade with an adjustable protective roller at the leading edge which determines the skin thickness taken (0.008–0.018 of an inch). If all the skin graft taken is not used during surgery, it can be wrapped in gauze soaked in sterile saline, put in a sterile container and kept in a fridge at 4° C for 2–3 weeks (Alderman, 1988; Coull, 1991).

The recipient area needs to be sufficiently vascular to support the metabolic needs of the graft and free from infection which causes breakdown of the fibrin adhesions between the bed and the graft. A graft will not take on bare bone, tendons, cartilage or nerves.

Within a few minutes of the graft being applied it begins to adhere to the recipient area with fibrin (Coull, 1991). The fibrin is infiltrated by fibroblasts which convert the fibrin clots into fibrous tissue and make the attachment firmer. After 24 hours the skin graft may appear pink and oedematous, but blood flow is not established until 3 days after grafting. Blood vessels bud from the split skin and these are reinforced by ingrowing vessels from the recipient area (Coull, 1991), reorganising the vascular pattern. It takes about 8 days for a mature complex of vessels to form and during this period nutritional needs are met by diffusion of the plasma which exudes from the recipient bed. Nerve endings grow into the skin graft from the edges and development of sensation to the area is slow (usually the thinner the graft, the quicker sensation develops).

After being applied, the skin graft will retain the colour and texture of the original site, together with its normal hair growth and function of sebaceous and sweat glands. Sensation usually returns in 1–5 months.

Indications for using a split skin graft

1. Restores skin cover.
2. Revascularises readily, therefore used extensively for covering large areas of full thickness burns.
3. May be expanded to cover large areas by meshing.
4. By ingrowth of nerves, moderate sensation is acquired.
5. Leaves enough dermis in the donor area for healing to take place within about 10 days.

Indications for not using a split skin graft

1. Contracts the surface area and is therefore unsuitable for use in areas such as the eyelids where contraction would result in ectropion (Kemble and Lamb, 1984).
2. If subjected to repeated trauma it tends to break down and ulcerate. Therefore it may be unsuitable for use on the hands of a manual worker.

Complications

A split skin graft may not take due to:

1. Poor blood supply.
2. Haematoma formation.
3. Shearing forces.
4. Applied onto bare tendons, cartilage, bone or nerves.
5. Infection, e.g. all groups of haemolytic streptococci.
6. Lyses epithelial cells, and pseudomonas aeruginosa which, by producing copius exudate, "floats" the graft off the recipient area.
7. Inadequately excised or debrided eschar.

Delayed skin graft

If the recipient area bleeds excessively during surgery, a delay of 24 hours allows time for the bleeding to stop before the graft is applied. Haemorrhage may prevent the graft from taking.

1. Procedure for the postoperative check of a split skin graft

A split skin graft is checked 3–7 days postoperatively according to instructions from the medical staff and the condition of the patient. Generally, the longer the graft is left undisturbed, the less risk there is of damaging the newly developing blood supply. However if infection is suspected or was present at the time of grafting a careful and early inspection to minimise skin loss is indicated.

See sections 1–5 in Chapter 1 for advice on procedures and sharps policy.

Equipment

Trolley
Sterile dressing pack
Sterile 20 ml syringe
1 pair of unsterile gloves
Bacteriological wound swab
Sterile gauze swabs
Sterile gauze applicators
Paraffin gauze
Sterile scissors
Sachet of normal saline and alcohol swab
Topical agents or wound care products (as appropriate)
Crepe bandage (of appropriate size)
Elasticated bandage (of appropriate size)
Elasticated bandage measure
Applicator
Adhesive tape
Disposal bag
Patient's prescription chart
Sharps box (optional)

Action	Rationale
Administer analgesia as prescribed approximately 30 minutes prior to the procedure and position the patient comfortably.	To minimise pain and discomfort for the patient.
Apply unsterile gloves and remove outer splints, bandages and outer dressings, e.g. Gamgee.	To minimise the risk of cross infection and allow access to the grafted area.
Discard dressings etc., into the disposal bag, remove gloves and wash hands.	To minimise the risk of cross infection.

Action	Rationale
Apply sterile gloves and remove the gauze as far as the paraffin gauze. This is done by applying gentle counterpressure to the paraffin gauze with one hand while peeling back the gauze with the other.	Pulling will lift the graft from its bed and cause damage to the site.
If the gauze is adherent, the area should be irrigated with normal saline. If the area is large then the patient should be bathed/showered.	Moistening the area will help to loosen adherent areas and any dried exudate (Alderman, 1988). The use of antiseptics should be avoided as they increase the inflammatory response (Brennan and Leaper, 1985). Bathing/showering facilities easy removal due to soaking.
Using forceps or a gloved hand, gently lift off the paraffin gauze while exerting gentle counterpressure onto the graft using forceps or a gloved finger.	To facilitate easy removal of the paraffin gauze and to prevent the graft from being pulled from its bed, using a shearing force. Forceps impair manual dexterity which can cause pain for the patient and tissue damage (Glide, 1992); gloves are preferable.
If the paraffin gauze is adherent, irrigate the area with saline.	To facilitate easy removal (Alderman, 1988).
Discard the gauze into the disposal bag, remove gloves, wash hands and apply second pair of sterile gloves.	To minimise the risk of cross infection.
If any exudate is present irrigate the graft with warmed normal saline using a syringe.	Irrigation with warmed saline or water may be sufficient to dislodge particles (Cutting, 1990; Stringer et al., 1983; Morison, 1989) and to remove debris while preventing pain and damage (caused by cleaning) to the ingrowth of capillaries (Thomas, 1990). Allows accurate assessment of the graft. Saline has no detrimental effect on granulation tissue (Brennan and Leaper, 1985). Warmed fluids help to prevent delays in wound healing caused by a drop in wound surface temperature (Turner, 1985; Lock, 1980).
Assess the graft for any skin loss, slough, haematoma formation, signs of infection, or overgranulation and report any abnormalities to the nurse in charge.	Haematoma formation and infection may cause the skin graft to fail (Coull, 1991). Extensive skin loss may require further skin grafting procedures or assessment of the wound for alternative treatment.

Action	Rationale
Areas that have "taken" will look pink/blue in colour and the graft will be adherent to the underlying tissue.	As the graft takes it will become pink/red and will not slip when rolling or during cleansing of the area (Coull, 1991).
Remove any staples on the advice of medical staff (Refer to section 3) and discard into the sharps box.	Staples are used to secure the split skin graft in position and promote immobilisation of the graft following surgery. To prevent injury and in accordance with unit sharps policy.
Using sharp scissors trim off any non-adherent graft.	The tissue of a non-adherent graft is dead and could encourage bacterial growth.
Snip any blisters on the graft and express the fluid by rolling a sterile gauze applicator soaked in saline over the area.	Allows the escape of fluid which if left, can lift the graft from its bed. The holes will allow any further collections of fluid to escape (Alderman, 1988).
Pustules should be expressed using the technique above for blisters and a bacteriological wound swab should be taken for culture and sensitivity. Label and send to the microbiology laboratory.	Culture and sensitivity will confirm the presence of any infection (Coull, 1991).
Irrigate the area with warmed normal saline using a syringe.	Irrigation is recommended to remove debris and dislodge particles (Cutting 1990; Stringer et al., 1983; Morison, 1989). Saline is recommended as antiseptics can be injurious to tissues (Brennan, Foster and Leaper, 1986).
	Warmed fluids help to prevent delays in wound healing caused by a drop in wound surface temperature (Turner, 1985; Lock, 1980).
Further treatment to areas where the graft has not taken will depend on the physical state of the area (Refer to section 2 below).	To promote healing and minimise complications.
Assess the wound and redress the graft using appropriate wound care products or agents and secondary dressing, e.g. a layer of sterile gauze and/or Gamgee (as appropriate).	To promote healing. Secondary dressings provide protection and absorb wound exudate (Gamgee, 1880).
Secure firmly with a bandage and adhesive tape (if appropriate).	Firm bandaging secures the dressing in place and is important in preventing slipping (Alderman, 1988), friction and shearing forces which will occur if the dressing/bandages are loose. It also provides support to the graft. Tape is preferable to pins for the safety of the patient.

Action	Rationale
Measure the graft area/limb using the elasticated bandage measure. Using the applicator apply a piece of elasticated bandage of the appropriate size.	The application of pressure helps to prevent the development of hypertrophic scarring. (Linares, Larson, Galstaun 1993; Scott-Ward 1991)
Ensure the patient is comfortable and the bandages are not too tight.	For the comfort of the patient.
Complete the appropriate nursing documentation noting the date of the next dressing.	To maintain an accurate record.
Record the wound care product on the patient's prescription chart.	In accordance with the unit policy/procedure for nurses prescribing wound care products.

2. Procedure for further treatment to areas where the split skin graft has not taken

Further treatment will depend on the physical state of the area.

See section 1–5 in Chapter 1 for advice on procedures.

Procedure for the treatment of sloughy areas

Equipment

Trolley
Sterile dressing pack
Sterile 20 ml syringe
1 pair of unsterile gloves
2 pairs of sterile gloves
Bacteriological wound swab
Sterile gauze swabs
Sterile gauze applicators
Paraffin gauze
Sterile scissors
Topical desloughing agent, e.g. hydrogels or enzymatic products
Barrier cream (of choice)
Crepe bandage (of appropriate size)
Adhesive tape
Elasticated bandage measure
Applicator
Elasticated bandage
Disposal bag
Patient's prescription chart

Action	Rationale
Administer analgesia as prescribed approximately 30 minutes prior to commencing the procedure and position the patient comfortably.	To minimise pain and discomfort for the patient.
Apply unsterile gloves and remove outer splints, bandages and outer dressings, e.g. Gamgee.	To minimise the risk of cross infection and allow access to the grafted area.
Discard dressings, etc. into the disposal bag, remove gloves and wash hands.	To minimise the risk of cross infection.
Apply sterile gloves and remove the dressing. This is done by applying gentle counterpressure with one hand while peeling back the gauze with the other.	Pulling will lift the graft from its bed and cause damage to the site.
If the dressing is adherent to the area it should be irrigated with normal saline. If the area is large then the patient should be bathed/showered.	Moistening the area will help to loosen adherent areas and any dried exudate (Alderman, 1988). The use of antiseptics should be avoided as they increase the inflammatory response (Brennan and Leaper, 1985). Bathing/showering facilitates easy removal due to soaking.
Using forceps or a gloved hand, gently lift off the dressing while exerting gentle counterpressure onto the graft.	To facilitate easy removal of the dressing and to prevent the graft from being pulled from its bed, using a shearing force. Gloves are preferable to forceps which inhibit dexterity, and cause pain and tissue damage (Glide, 1992).
If the dressing is adherent, irrigate the area with warmed saline.	To facilitate easy removal of the dressing and to minimise the risk of damage to the wound bed (Morison, 1989; Thomas, 1990).
Discard the dressings into the disposal bag, remove gloves, wash hands and apply second pair of sterile gloves.	To minimise the risk of cross infection.
Assess the graft for any skin loss, slough, haematoma formation, signs of infection or overgranulation and report any abnormalities to the nurse in charge.	Haematoma formation and infection may cause skin loss (Coull, 1991). Extensive skin loss may require further skin grafting procedures or assessment of the wound for alternative treatment.
Take a bacteriological wound swab if wound appears red, inflamed or malodorous. Label and send to the microbiology laboratory for culture and sensitivity.	To allow for prompt and appropriate treatment if infection is present. For documentation and to assist with planning the appropriate treatment.
Areas that have "taken" will look pink/blue in colour and the graft will be adherent to the underlying tissue.	As the graft takes it will become pink/red and will not slip during cleansing of the area (Coull, 1991).

Action	Rationale
Using sharp scissors trim off any non-adherent graft.	The tissue is dead and could encourage bacterial growth (Lawrence, 1989).
Snip any blisters on the graft and express the fluid by rolling a sterile gauze applicator soaked in saline over the area.	Allows the escape of fluid which, if left, can lift the graft from its bed. The hole(s) will allow any further collections of fluid to escape (Alderman, 1988).
If any exudate or loose dead tissue is present, irrigate the area with warmed saline using a syringe.	To remove debris which is likely to delay healing and act as a focus for infection (Morison, 1989) while preventing damage caused by cleaning to the ingrowth of capillaries. Irrigation is effective and less harmful to the wound in the long term (Thomas, 1990). Warmed fluids help prevent delays in wound healing caused by a drop in wound surface temperature (Turner, 1985; Lock, 1980). Allows accurate assessment of the area.
Using forceps lift up any loose slough and with sterile scissors cut off as close to the skin as possible.	Slough can be a focus for bacterial growth (Lawrence, 1989). It prolongs the inflammatory stage and will delay healing.
Any remaining slough should be treated with a desloughing agent which is not chemically damaging. Contact with the graft should be avoided.	Grafted tissue is fragile.
Apply a barrier cream to the healthy tissue and surrounding skin.	Protects the healthy tissue from damage and maceration.
Apply the desloughing or enzymatic agent, e.g. Intrasite, Aserbine cream Varidase, to the sloughy areas being treated only.	To allow the desloughing or enzymatic agent to act only on the slough and not destroy the surrounding tissue.
If using a hydrogel ensure a satisfactory margin around the wound.	Hydrogels prevent loss of water vapour from the surface of the wound and effectively rehydrate dead tissue which can then be removed by autolysis (Thomas, 1994 b).
	Intrasite is advocated for the treatment of dry sloughy or necrotic wounds promoting debridement by facilitating rehydration and autolysis of dead tissue (Thomas, 1994 a).
	Aserbine cream is a combination of malic, benzoic and salicylic acid. It is water soluble and has the ability to break down necrotic tissue (de Kock and van der Merwe, 1987).
	Varidase is indicated for cleansing and desloughing of necrotic and infected wounds (Morgan 1992).

Action	Rationale
Redress the wound using appropriate topical agents and secondary dressings, e.g. a layer of sterile gauze and/or Gamgee.	To promote healing. Gauze and/or Gamgee provide protection and absorb wound exudate (Gamgee, 1880).
Secure firmly with a bandage and adhesive tape.	Firm bandaging secures the dressing in place and is important in preventing friction and shearing forces which will occur if the dressing/bandages are loose. It also provides support to the graft. Tape is preferable to pins for the safety of the patient.
Measure the grafted area/limb using appropriate measure. Using the applicator, apply a piece of elasticated bandage of the appropriate size.	The application of pressure helps to prevent the development of hypertrophic scarring. (Scott-Ward 1991: Linares, Larson, Galstaun 1993)
Ensure the patient is comfortable and the bandages are not too tight.	For the comfort of the patient.
Complete the appropriate nursing documentation noting the date of the next dressing.	To maintain an accurate record.
Record the wound care product on the patient's prescription chart.	In accordance with the unit policy/procedure for nurses prescribing wound care products.

Procedure for the treatment of overgranulation tissue

Overgranulation tissue is recognised by pink/red lumps. It can be caused by a reaction to infection or a prolonged inflammatory response. The aim is to reduce the granulations.

See sections 1–5 in Chapter 1 for advice on procedures.

Equipment

Trolley
Sterile dressing pack
Sterile 20 ml syringe
1 pair of unsterile gloves
2 pairs of sterile gloves
Sterile gauze swabs
Paraffin gauze
Sterile scissors
Topical agents (of choice)
Irrigation catheter and spigot (optional)
Crepe bandage (of appropriate size)

Adhesive tape
Elasticated bandage measure
Elasticated bandage (of appropriate size)
Disposal bag
Patient's prescription chart.

Action	Rationale
Administer analgesia as prescribed approximately 20 minites prior to commencing the procedure and position the patient comfortably.	To minimise pain and discomfort for the patient.
Apply unsterile gloves and remove outer splints, bandages and outer dressings, e.g. Gamgee	To minimise the risk of cross infection and allow access to the grafted area.
Discard dressings into the disposal bag, remove gloves and wash hands.	To minimise the risk of cross infection.
Apply sterile gloves and remove the dressing. This is done by applying gentle counterpressure with one hand while peeling back the gauze with the other.	Pulling will lift the graft from its bed and cause damage to the site.
If the gauze is adherent to the area it should be irrigated with normal saline. If the area is large then the patient should be bathed/showered.	Moistening the area will help to loosen adherent areas and any dried exudate (Alderman, 1988). The use of antiseptics should be avoided as they increase the inflammatory response (Brennan and Leaper, 1985). Bathing/showering facilitates easy removal due to soaking.
Using forceps or a gloved hand, gently lift off the dressing while exerting gentle counterpressure onto the graft using forceps or a gloved finger.	To facilitate easy removal of the dressing and to prevent the graft from being pulled from its bed, using a shearing force. Gloves are preferable to forceps which inhibit dexterity, and cause pain and tissue damage (Glide, 1992).
If the dressing is adherent, irrigate the area with warmed saline.	To facilitate easy removal of the dressing and to minimise the risk of damage to the wound bed (Morison, 1989; Thomas, 1990).
Discard the dressings into the disposal bag, remove gloves, wash hands and apply second pair of sterile gloves.	To minimise the risk of cross infection.

Action	Rationale
If any exudate is present irrigate the graft with warmed normal saline using a syringe.	To remove debris which is likely to delay healing and act as a focus for infection (Morison, 1989) while preventing damage to the ingrowth of capillaries caused by cleaning (Alderman, 1988). Irrigation is effective and less harmful to the wound in the long term (Thomas, 1990). Warmed fluids help prevent delays in wound healing caused by a drop in wound surface temperature (Turner, 1985; Lock, 1980).
Assess the graft for any skin loss, slough, haematoma formation, signs of infection, or overgranulation and report any abnormalities to the nurse in charge.	Haematoma formation and infection may cause skin loss (Coull, 1991). Burns at the granulating phase of healing are prone to healing in an uneven sequence causing overgranulation which appears as red, raw, raised bumpy patches (Orr and Hain, 1994). Extensive skin loss may require further skin grafting procedures or assessment of the wound for alternative treatment.
Areas that have "taken" will look pink/blue in colour and the graft will be adherent to the underlying tissue.	For documentation and to assist with planning the appropriate treatment. As the graft takes it will become pink/red and will not slip during cleansing of the area (Coull, 1991).
Using sharp scissors trim off any non-adherent graft.	The tissue is dead and could encourage bacterial growth (Lawrence, 1989).
If there are only a few small overgranulations apply an anti-inflammatory antibacterial cream directly to them.	This type of product will reduce the inflammatory response and thus the overgranulation.
If the overgranulations are larger and more widespread apply one layer of paraffin gauze to the area with hypertonic saline (20%) soaked gauzed directly on top.	Paraffin gauze will prevent the saline-soaked gauze from adhering to the graft if it dries out (Thomas, 1994 c). Hypertonic saline draws fluid from the granulation tissue by osmosis and reduces the size of the granulations.
Insert a catheter with a spigot end into the gauze. Irrigate 4–6 hourly (or change the wet soaks 3–4 times daily).	Insertion of a catheter with a spigot provides access for continual irrigation to keep the gauze moist.
Apply gauze and Gamgee, secure with a bandage and adhesive tape.	To absorb fluid and to prevent outer dressings becoming moist. Bandages secure the dressing in place and reduce friction and shearing forces which will occur if the dressing/ bandages are loose. Tape is preferable to pins for safety of the patient.

Action	Rationale
Measure the grafted area/limb using the appropriate measure. Using the applicator apply a piece of elasticated bandage of the appropriate size.	The application of pressure helps to prevent the development of hypertrophic scarring. (Scott-Ward 1991: Linares, Larson, Galstaun 1993)
Ensure the patient is comfortable and the bandages are not too tight.	For the comfort of the patient.
Complete the appropriate documentation and assess the wound in 12–24 hours.	To maintain an accurate record and to assess the effectiveness of the treatment.
Record the wound care product on the patient's prescription chart.	In accordance with unit policy/procedure for nurses prescribing wound care products.

Procedure for the treatment of infected areas

Burns frequently become colonised with haemolytic streptococcus and pseudomonas. See sections 1–5 in Chapter 1 for advice on procedures.

Equipment

Trolley
Sterile dressing pack
Sterile 20 ml syringe
1 pair of unsterile gloves
2 pairs of sterile gloves
Sterile gauze swabs
Sterile gauze applicators
Bacteriological wound swab
Paraffin gauze
Sterile scissors
Topical antibacterial or medicated products
Irrigation catheter and spigot (optional)
Crepe bandage (of appropriate size)
Adhesive tape
Elasticated bandage measure
Applicator
Elasticated bandage (of appropriate size)
Disposal bag
Patient's prescription chart

Action	Rationale
Administer analgesia as prescribed approximately 30 minutes prior to commencing the procedure and position the patient comfortably.	To minimise pain and discomfort for the patient.
Apply unsterile gloves and remove outer splints, bandages and outer dressings, e.g. Gamgee.	To minimise the risk of cross infection and allow access to the grafted area.
Discard dressings, etc. into the disposal bag, remove gloves and wash hands.	To minimise the risk of cross infection.
Apply sterile gloves and remove the dressing. This is done by applying gentle counterpressure with one hand while peeling back the gauze with the other.	Pulling will lift the graft from its bed and cause damage to the site.
If the dressing is adherent to the area it should be irrigated with normal saline. If the area is large then the patient should be bathed/showered.	Moistening the area will help to loosen adherent areas and any dried exudate (Alderman, 1988). The use of antiseptics should be avoided as they increase the inflammatory response (Brennan and Leaper, 1985). Bathing/showering facilitates easy removal due to soaking.
Using forceps or a gloved hand, gently lift off the dressing while exerting gentle counterpressure onto the graft using forceps or a gloved finger.	To facilitate easy removal of the dressing and to prevent the graft from being pulled from its bed, using a shearing force. Gloves are preferable to forceps which inhibit dexterity and may cause pain for the patient and tissue damage (Glide, 1992).
If the dressing is adherent, irrigate the area with warmed saline.	To facilitate easy removal of the dressing and to minimise the risk of damage to the wound bed (Morison, 1989; Thomas, 1990).
Discard the dressings into the disposal bag, remove gloves, wash hands and apply second pair of sterile gloves.	To minimise the risk of cross infection.
If any exudate or loose dead tissue is present irrigate the area with warmed saline using a syringe.	To remove debris which is likely to delay healing and act as a focus for infection (Morison, 1989) while preventing damage to the ingrowth of capillaries caused by cleaning (Alderman, 1988). Irrigation is effective and less harmful to the wound in the long term (Thomas, 1990). Warmed fluids help prevent delays in wound healing caused by a drop in wound surface temperature (Turner, 1985; Lock, 1980).

Action	Rationale
Assess the graft for any skin loss, slough, haematoma formation, signs of infection or overgranulation and report any abnormalities to the nurse in charge.	Haematoma formation and infection may cause skin loss. Extensive skin loss may require further skin grafting procedures or assessment of the wound for alternative treatment. For documentation and to assist with planning the appropriate treatment.
Areas that have "taken" will look pink/blue in colour and the graft will be adherent to the underlying tissue.	As the graft takes it will become pink/red and will not slip during cleansing of the area (Coull, 1991).
Using sharp scissors trim off any non-adherent graft.	The tissue is dead and could encourage bacterial growth (Lawrence, 1989).
Pustules should be expressed by rolling a sterile gauze applicator soaked in saline over the area and a bacteriological wound swab should be taken for culture and sensitivity. Label and send to the microbiology laboratory.	Culture and sensitivity allows prompt and accurate treatment if infection is present.
Irrigate the area with warmed saline using a syringe. or	To remove debris (Morison, 1989; Thomas, 1990). Warmed fluids help prevent delays in wound healing caused by a drop in wound surface temperature (Turner, 1985; Lock, 1980).
Irrigate the area with aqueous Povidone Iodine aqueous solution (10%).	This is a broad spectrum antiseptic. Research shows that it does not reduce healing times (Gilmore, Vistines and Stroken, 1977).
Apply an antibacterial product, e.g. Silver Sulphadiazine or Betadine cream, Iodoflex, or Iodosorb ointment, directly to the infected area.	Infection is a threat to the graft, causing skin loss. Treatment will improve the chance of healing or "take" when the area is regrafted. A reduction in the number of surface organisms will lower the risk of septicaemia.
	Betadine is effective against both gram-negative and gram-positive bacterial, fungi, yeasts, viruses and protozoa (McKnight, 1965; Copeland, 1972; de Kock and van der Merwe, 1987).
	Iodoflex is a medicated dressing of polysaccharide beads which releases iodine as the beads take up fluid, and imparts antibacterial properties to the wound (Thomas, 1994 d).

Action	Rationale
	Iodosorb ointment acts as Iodoflex releasing iodine and imparting antibacterial properties (Thomas, 1994 e).
Redress the graft using appropriate topical agents, and secondary dressing, e.g. a layer of sterile gauze and/or Gamgee.	To promote healing. Gauze and/or Gamgee provide protection and absorb wound exudate.
Secure firmly with a bandage and adhesive tape.	Firm bandaging secures the dressing in place and is important in preventing friction and shearing forces which will occur if the dressing/bandages are loose. It also provides support to the graft. Tape is preferable to pins for the safety of the patient.
Measure the grafted area/limb using the appropriate measure. Using the applicator, apply a piece of elasticated bandage of the appropriate size.	The application of pressure helps to prevent the development of hypertrophic scarring. (Scott-Ward 1991: Linares, Larson, Galstaun 1993)
Ensure the patient is comfortable and the bandages are not too tight.	For the comfort of the patient.
If the area is affected by pseudomonas:	The growth of this organism is inhibited by lowering the pH level of the tissue.
– Apply one layer of paraffin gauze to the area with gauze soaked in 1% acetic acid on top.	To prevent the gauze from adhering to the graft. Allows anti-bacterial activity to the whole area.
– Insert a catheter with a spigot end into the gauze. Irrigate 4–6 hourly (or change the wet soaks 3–4 times daily).	Prevents the soaks from drying out. Frequent treatment will reduce multiplication of micro-organisms.
Apply gauze and Gamgee, secure with a bandage and adhesive tape.	To absorb fluid and prevent the outer dressings becoming moist. Bandages secure the dressing in place. Tape is preferable to pins for the safety of the patient.
Measure the grafted area/limb using the appropriate measure. Using the applicator apply a piece of elasticated bandage of the appropriate size.	The application of pressure helps to prevent the development of hypertrophic scarring. (Scott-Ward 1991: Linares, Larson, Galstaun 1993)
Ensure the patient is comfortable and the bandages are not too tight.	For the comfort of the patient.
Complete the appropriate nursing documentation and assess the wound in 24 hours. Record the wound care product on the patient's prescription chart.	To maintain an accurate record and to assess the effectiveness of the treatment. In accordance with unit policy/procedure for nurses prescribing wound care products.

3. Procedure for removal of staples from a split skin graft

Skin staples are used in abdominal, gynaecological, orthopaedic and thoracic surgery for closure of skin, and can also be applied directly over bone or viscera. Additional uses include closure of scalp incisions, scalp flap haemostasis, skin grafts, and plastic and reconstructive surgery.

The staples are made of stainless steel wire and are approximately 4.8–6.5 mm wide and 3.4–3.6 mm high (when closed) and are used to secure split skin grafts in position and promote immobilisation of the graft following surgery.

The staples are usually removed 3–7 days postoperatively on the advice of the medical staff and in conjunction with the procedure for a post-operative check of a split skin graft.

See sections 1–5 in Chapter 1 for advice on procedures

Equipment

Trolley
Sterile dressing pack
Sterile 20 ml syringe
1 pair of unsterile gloves
2 pairs of sterile gloves
Bacteriological wound swab
Sterile gauze swabs
Gamgee
Sterile gauze applicators
Wound dressing (of choice)
Sterile scissors
Sterile auto-suture staple remover
Sachet of normal saline and alcohol swab
Topical agents wound care product (of choice)
Crepe bandage (of appropriate size)
Adhesive tape
Disposal bag
Sharps box
Patient's prescription chart

Action	Rationale
Administer analgesia as prescribed approximately 30 minutes prior to commencing the procedure and position the patient comfortably.	To minimise pain and discomfort for the patient.
Apply unsterile gloves and remove outer splints, bandages and outer dressings, e.g. Gamgee.	To minimise the risk of cross infection and allow access to the grafted area.

Action	Rationale
Discard dressings, etc. into the disposal bag, remove gloves and wash hands.	To minimise the risk of cross infection.
Apply sterile gloves and remove the gauze as far as the paraffin gauze. This is done by applying gentle counterpressure to the dressing with one hand while peeling back the gauze with the other.	Pulling will lift the graft from its bed and cause damage to the site.
If the gauze is adherent to the area it should be irrigated with normal saline. If the area is large then the patient should be bathed/showered.	Moistening the area will help to loosen adherent areas and any dried exudate (Alderman, 1988). The use of antiseptics should be avoided as they increase the inflammatory response (Brennan and Leaper, 1985). Bathing/showering facilitates easy removal due to soaking.
Using forceps or a gloved hand, gently lift off the dressing while exerting gentle counterpressure onto the graft.	To facilitate easy removal of the dressing and to prevent the graft from being pulled from its bed, using a shearing force. Gloves are preferable to forceps which impair manual dexterity which can cause pain for the patient and tissue damage (Glide, 1992).
If the dressing is adherent, irrigate the area with saline.	To facilitate easy removal (Alderman, 1988).
Discard the dressings into the disposal bag, remove gloves, wash hands and apply second pair of sterile gloves.	To minimise the risk of cross infection.
If any exudate is present irrigate the graft with warmed normal saline using a syringe.	Irrigation with warmed saline or water using a syringe may be sufficient to dislodge particles (Cutting, 1990; Stringer et al., 1983; Morison, 1989) and to remove debris while preventing pain and damage to the ingrowth of capillaries caused by cleaning (Thomas, 1990). Allows accurate assessment of the graft. Saline has no detrimental effect on granulation tissue (Brennan and Leaper, 1985).
	Warmed fluids help prevent delays in wound healing caused by a drop in wound surface temperature (Turner, 1985; Lock, 1980).
Assess the graft for any skin loss, slough, haematoma formation, signs of infection or overgranulation and report any abnormalities to the nurse in charge.	Haematoma formation and infection may cause skin loss (Coull, 1991). Extensive skin loss may require further skin grafting procedures or assessment of the wound for alternative treatment. For documentation and to assist with planning the appropriate treatment.

Action	Rationale
Areas that have "taken" will look pink/blue in colour and the graft will be adherent to the underlying tissue.	As the graft takes it will become pink/red and will not slip when rolling or during cleansing of the area (Coull, 1991).
Open the handles of the staple remover.	To open the jaws of the staple remover.
Gently slip the lower jaws of the staple remover under the staple and rest the upper jaw on top of the staple (see Figure 24.2).	To ensure the correct position of the auto-suture remover.
Ensure both tips are under the staple before proceeding.	To minimise trauma to the skin graft and patient discomfort when the staple is removed.
Close the handles to unbend the staple (see Figure 24.3)	To facilitate easy removal of the staple.
Gently but firmly lift the staple straight up (see Figure 24.4)	To minimise trauma to the skin graft.
Dispose of the staple into the sharps box.	To prevent injury and in accordance with the unit sharps policy.
Continue to remove the staples (as above) around the circumference and across the surface area of the skin graft.	To remove all the staples.
Check carefully for any further staples.	To avoid any staples being left *in situ*.
Where an excessive number of staples have been used, the medical staff may recommend an X-ray of the skin graft site.	Staples can become buried in tissue, an X-ray will identify the site of any hidden staples. Prompt removal will minimise the risk of future irritation or breakdown of the skin graft.
Using sharp scissors trim off any non-adherent graft.	The tissue of a non-adherent graft is dead and could encourage bacterial growth.
Snip any blisters from the graft and express the fluid by rolling a sterile gauze applicator soaked in saline over the area.	Allows the escape of fluid which, if left, could lift the graft from its bed. The hole(s) will allow any further collections of fluid to escape (Alderman, 1988).
Pustules should be expressed using the technique above for blisters and a bacteriological wound swab should be taken for culture and sensitivity. Label and send to the microbiology laboratory.	Culture and sensitivity will confirm the presence of any infection (Coull, 1991). Allows for prompt and appropriate treatment to be carried out.

Action	Rationale
Irrigate the area with warmed normal saline using a syringe.	To remove debris and dislodge particles (Cutting, 1990; Stringer et al., 1983; Morison, 1989). Warmed fluids help prevent delays in wound healing caused by a drop in wound surface temperature (Turner, 1985; Lock, 1980). Saline is preferable to antiseptics (Brennan, Foster and Leaper, 1986).
Further treatment to areas where the graft has not taken will depend on the physical state of the area (see section 2 above).	To promote healing and minimise complications.
Assess the wound and redress the graft using appropriate wound care products or topical agents and secondary dressings, e.g. a layer of sterile gauze and/or Gamgee (as appropriate).	To promote healing. Gauze and/or Gamgee provide protection and absorb wound exudate (Gamgee, 1880).
Secure firmly with a bandage and adhesive tape (if appropriate).	Firm bandaging secures the dressing in place and helps to prevent friction and shearing forces which will occur if the dressing/bandages are loose. It also provides support to the graft. Tape is preferable to pins for the safety of the patient.
Measure the grafted area/limb using the appropriate measure. Using the applicator, apply a piece of elasticated bandage of the appropriate size.	The application of pressure helps to prevent the development of hypertrophic scarring. (Scott-Ward 1991: Linares, Larson, Galstaun 1993)
Ensure the patient is comfortable and the bandages are not too tight.	For the comfort of the patient.
Complete the appropriate nursing documentation and record the type of wound care product used on the patient's prescription chart.	To maintain an accurate record. In accordance with unit policy/procedure for nurses prescribing wound care products.

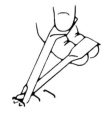
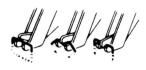

EXTRACTED
STAPLE

Figure 24.2 *Lower the jaws of the staple remover under the staple and rest the upper jaws on top of the staple.*
Figure 24.3 *Close the handles to unbend the staple.* Figure 24.4 *An extracted staple.*

4. Procedure for the application of a delayed split skin graft

Delayed split skin grafting is used if the recipient area bleeds excessively during surgery and application of a skin graft at that time is not possible. It is usually performed 24–48 hours postoperatively when bleeding has subsided. This procedure is part of an expanded role for nurses on the Burns Unit.

See sections 1–5 in Chapter 1 for advice on procedures.

Equipment

Trolley
Sterile towels (optional)
Sterile dressing pack (with sterile scissors)
Sterile 50 ml syringe
1 pair of sterile gloves
Sterile field
Patient's stored skin (not more than 3 weeks old)
Bottle of sterile normal saline
Paraffin gauze or wound dressing (of choice)
Sterile gauze
Sterile gauze applicators
Gamgee
Crepe bandage (of appropriate size)
Adhesive tape
Sterile towels (optional)
1 pair of unsterile gloves
Bacteriological wound swab (optional)
Disposal bag
Patient's prescription chart

Action	Rationale
Check the patient's previous wound swab results from the recipient area. If growing haemolytic streptococcus, postpone procedure until three clear wound swabs have been obtained and isolate the patient in a single room.	Haemolytic streptococcus lyses epithelial cells causing loss of skin graft. Three clear swabs indicate the patient is clear of infection. Isolation is recommended to minimise the risk of cross infection by contact and airborne routes.
Administer analgesia as prescribed 30 minutes prior to commencing the procedure and position the patient comfortably.	To minimise pain and discomfort for the patient.
Apply unsterile gloves and remove the outer dressings of the recipient area.	To minimise the risk of cross infection and allow access to the wound site.

Action	Rationale
If the dressing is adherent the area should be irrigated with normal saline using a syringe.	Pulling/friction will cause damage to the ingrowing capillaries. Moistening the area helps to loosen adherent tissue (Alderman, 1988).
Discard the dressings into the disposal bag, remove gloves and wash hands.	To minimise the risk of cross infection.
Apply sterile gloves and position the sterile field under the area to be grafted.	To minimise the risk of cross infection. To prevent soiling of linen and to maintain a sterile field.
If the wound bed appears cellulitic, infected and/or if slough is present do not apply the skin graft and report to the nurse in charge.	For early detection of infection which may cause loss of graft.
Take a bacteriological wound swab. Label and send to the microbiology laboratory for culture and sensitivity. Redress the wound with the appropriate wound dressing of choice.	Culture and sensitivity allows for suitable treatment to be instigated.
If the wound appears healthy with a good blood supply, irrigate with warmed sterile normal saline and a syringe ensuring all post-operative haematomas have been removed and there are no bleeding points.	The use of antiseptics should be avoided as they increase the inflammatory response (Brennan and Leaper, 1985). Warmed fluids help prevent delays in wound healing caused by a drop in wound surface temperature (Turner, 1985; Lock, 1980). Irrigation is preferable to cleaning in preventing damage to new epithelial cells (Cutting, 1990; Stringer et al., 1983; Morison, 1989). Haematomas reduce adherence of the skin graft to the wound bed.
Check the container holds the correct patient's skin and the date has not expired.	To ensure the patient receives their own skin. Split thickness skin can be stored at 4°C for up to 3 weeks (Coull, 1991).
Remove the skin from the container and unwrap it from the sterile soaked saline gauze.	To facilitate access to skin. Skin needs to be kept moist during storage to prevent it from drying out.
Assess the size of the area to receive a skin graft and if possible apply the skin in one piece.	To produce a better cosmetic result.
If the skin is not meshed, use the sterile scissors to make small cuts randomly across the skin graft surface.	To allow exudate to pass through the holes. If exudate collects beneath the graft it will cause the graft to lift off.

Action	Rationale
Cut the required size of skin and leave attached to the paraffin gauze.	Leaving the skin on the paraffin gauze facilitates easy application.
Apply the skin (shiny side down) onto the recipient area. Overlap the edges slightly onto the good skin or where two or more pieces of graft meet.	The skin will not take if applied upside down.
Remove the paraffin gauze backing with forceps.	Removing the paraffin gauze facilitates easy viewing of the graft.
Using the forceps smooth the skin over the recipient area and trim the split skin graft to shape, slightly overlapping the defect.	To remove any bubbles or creases, to express out any air and serous fluid (Coull, 1991) and to ensure the graft is in contact with the recipient area. The skin must lie flush with the recipient bed and overlap the defect as the skin will shrink away from the edges as it 'takes' (Coull, 1991).
Gently roll sterile gauze applicators soaked in saline across the applied skin graft from one side to the other.	To express any serous fluid and or blood from under the graft which may cause it to lift from its bed and prevent it from 'taking' (Coull, 1991). Gauze is preferable to cotton wool as there is less likelihood of the filaments of fibre sticking to the wound edges.
If the delayed split skin graft is to be left exposed:	Exposed grafts are more easily observed and therefore complications can be detected early (Coull, 1991). However, the grafts are not protected from removal, e.g. by shearing forces.
− Check graft hourly.	To prevent serous fluid from collecting under the graft.
− Clean as necessary by gently rolling sterile gauze applicators soaked in saline from the centre outwards.	To prevent serous fluid from collecting under the graft.
− If blood or serum collects in the centre of the graft as a blister, snip a small hole in the skin with sterile sharp scissors and express the fluid.	To prevent serous fluid from collecting under the graft, and lifting the skin from the recipient area.
− Immobilise the graft site for 3–5 days.	To prevent accidental removal of the skin graft.
− If the grafted area will be covered by bed linen, apply a frame covered in sterile towels under the bed clothes until the graft is stable.	To protect the grafted area from being sheared off by bed linen.

Action	Rationale
If the graft is to be dressed:	Dressed grafts are protected. Padding and pressure from the dressing can help to expel any blistering (Coull, 1991) and to prevent serous fluid from collecting under the graft.
– Apply two layers of paraffin gauze to the skin graft.	To provide a non-adherent dressing.
– Cover with saline soaked gauze.	To provide a moist environment to facilitate healing and prevent the skin graft from drying out.
– Apply further layers of dry gauze and Gamgee.	To absorb any exudate.
– Apply crepe bandage firmly and secure with adhesive tape.	The application of pressure will help prevent fluid from collecting beneath the graft.
– Leave the dressing in place and immobilise the area for 3–5 days unless otherwise requested by the medical staff. (If lower limbs have been grafted, the patient should remain non-weight bearing for 5–7 days.)	To prevent movement of and any stress to the graft (Coull, 1991) and allow time for the skin graft to adhere and stabilise. Inadequate vascular supply to the recipient bed will compromise the graft. Also early and inappropriate movement of the grafted area will damage the delicate capillaries growing from the recipient bed into the grafted skin (Coull, 1991).
– Elevate grafted limbs on pillows or in slings and sit the patient upright well supported by pillows if graft is to the face or scalp.	To reduce oedema and maintain gravitational stasis.
Record in the appropriate nursing documentation. Record the type of wound care products used on the patient's prescription chart.	To maintain an accurate record. In accordance with unit policy/procedure for nurses prescribing wound care products.

5. Procedure for the aftercare of a split skin graft

The aim of aftercare of skin grafts is to minimise scar formation, reduce the need for further surgery and to produce a better cosmetic result. Aftercare may be carried out by any carer who has had instruction on what should be done and why, or may be carried out by the patient him or herself. Aftercare also gives the patient an opportunity to discuss with the carer his or her fears and anxieties about altered body image.

See section 1 in Chapter 1 for advice on procedures.

Equipment

Trolley or patient's bedside table
1 pair of unsterile gloves
Bowl of warm water
Patient's flannel or disposable wipes
Mild unscented soap
Towel
Non-perfumed, oil-based, moisturising cream
Elasticated bandage measure
Elasticated bandage (of appropriate size) or patient's own pressure garment
Applicator
Patient's prescription chart

Action	Rationale
Ensure the patient is in a comfortable position, in a quiet, private area.	This should help the patient to relax and be comfortable.
Wash hands and apply unsterile gloves.	For the protection of the nurse and to minimise the risk of cross infection.
Wash the grafted area(s) with the non-perfumed soap and flannel or wipes.	A perfumed soap could irritate the skin. Soaping helps to prevent a build up of cream which could lead to blocked pores.
Rinse the area(s) with clean water and pat dry with a towel, do not rub.	Rubbing can cause a breakdown of the skin as the epithelium is immature and delicate.
Massage the grafted area(s) with the non-perfumed oil-based cream until all the cream has been completely absorbed.	Massaging helps to break down the irregular pattern formation of collagen fibres in the scar tissue. Massaging is also stress relieving. Oil-based cream will prevent dryness caused by a lack of sebum in the skin due to damaged sebaceous glands.
Remove gloves and wash hands	
Encourage the patient to partake in his or her own aftercare as much as possible.	To promote independence. Touching the grafted area will help the patient to accept and come to terms with the scarring.
Measure the grafted area(s)/limb with the measure and choose the appropriate sized piece of elasticated bandage to cover the area. or Apply the patient's own pressure garment.	To ensure the correct size for the patient. Pressure is most readily maintained by elasticated garments. The application of pressure helps to prevent the development of hypertrophic scarring (Scott-Ward 1991; Linares, Larson, Galstaun 1993).

Action	Rationale
Explain to the patient why the elasticated bandage/garment must be worn 24 hours a day and should only be removed for washing and creaming during the next 6–24 months.	Mechanical pressure must be continued until the scar maturation process is completed.
	The severity of hypertrophic scarring can be reduced or even prevented by the use of tailored elastic pressure garments (Boore, Champion, and Ferguson, 1987).
Ensure the patient is left feeling comfortable and allow time for discussion about altered body image.	To provide a safe environment. Open communication will help the patient to come to terms with his or her new appearance.
Repeat the above aftercare procedures three times a day.	This will result in scarring which is flatter, paler, suppler and has a better cosmetic appearance.
If the patient complains of itching administer oral antihistamine tablets/syrup as prescribed and encourage the patient not to scratch the area. If warm, aim to keep the area cool and advise the patient to wear cotton clothes.	Itching is a frustrating effect of scarring (Cooper and Fenton 1996). Exact cause is unknown but antihistamine preparations relieve the itching and maintain the comfort of the patient. Scratching will cause damage to the new epithelial cells.

References

Alderman C (1988) Reconstructive approach. Nursing Standard. 7 May: 24–5.

Boore JRP, Champion R, Ferguson MC (1987) Nursing the Physically Ill Adult. Edinburgh: Churchill Livingstone.

Brennan SS, Foster ME, Leaper DJ (1986) Antiseptic toxicity in wounds healing by secondary intention. Journal of Hospital Infection 8: 263–7.

Brennan SS, Leaper DJ (1985) The effects of antiseptics on the healing wound. British Journal of Surgery. 72: 780–82.

Cooper R, Fenton O (1996) Disfigurement and disablement. In Settle JAD, Burns Management. Edinburgh: Churchill Livingstone.

Copeland CE (1972) The use of topical povidone iodine in the treatment of 30 burn patients. In Polk HC, Ehrenkranz NJ, (Eds). Proceedings for a Symposium of Therapeutic Advances and New Clinical Implications. Medical and Surgical Antiseptics with Betadine Microbicides. At the University of Miami, School of Medicine, April 1971. Yonkers N Y: The Purdue Frederick Co. p 129.

Coull A (1991) Making sense of split skin grafts. Nursing Times 87 (27): 54–5.

Cutting K (1990) Wound cleansing. Surgical Nurse 3 (3): 4–8.

de Kock M, van der Merwe AE (1987) A study to assess the effects of a new Betadine cream formulation compared to a standard treatment regimen for burns. Burns Journal 13 (1): 69–74.

Gamgee JS (1880) Absorbent and medical surgical dressings. Lancet 1: 127.

Gilmore O, Vistines L, Stroken A (1977) A study of the effect of povidone iodine on wound healing. Postgraduate Medical Journal 53: 122–5.

Glide S (1992) Cleaning choices. Nursing Times 88 (19): 74–8.

Kemble JV, Lamb BE (1984) Plastic Surgery and Burns Nursing. London: Bailliére Tindall.

Lawrence JC (1989) Management of burns. The Dressing Times 2 (3): 1–4.

Linares HA, Larson DL, Galstaun BA (1993) Historical notes on the use of pressure in the treatment of hypertrophic scars or Keloids. Burns Journal 19: 17–21.

Lock P (1980) Proceedings of the Symposium in Wound Healing. Gothenburg: Linden and Sonner.

McKnight AG (1965) A clinical trial of Povidone iodine in the treatment of chronic leg ulcers. Practitioner 195: 230.

Morgan DA (1992) Formulary of Wound Management Products (5th Ed) Chichester: Media Medica Publications Ltd. p.49.

Morison M (1989) Wound cleansing, which solution? Professional Nurse. February: 220–5.

Orr J, Hain T (1994) Burn wound management: an overview. Professional Nurse December: 153–6.

Scott-Ward R (1991) Pressure therapy for the control of hypertropic scar formation after burn injury. A history and review. Journal of Burn Care and Rehabilitation 12(3): 257–61.

Stringer M et al. (1983) Antiseptics and the casualty wound. Journal of Hospital Infection 4: 410–13.

Thomas S (1990) Wound Management and the Dressings. London: Pharmaceutical Press.

Thomas S (1994 a) Intrasite Gel. In Thomas S, (Ed) Handbook of Wound Dressings (1994 Edition) London: MacMillan Ltd. pp 90–1.

Thomas S (1994 b) Granuflex. In Thomas S, (Ed) Handbook of Wound Dressings (1994 Edition) London: MacMillan Ltd. pp 74–5.

Thomas S (1994 c) Jelonet. In Thomas S, (Ed) Handbook of Wound Dressings (1994 Edition) London: MacMillan Ltd. pp 98–9.

Thomas S (1994 d) Iodoflex. In Thomas S, (Ed) Handbook of Wound Dressings (1994 Edition) London: MacMillan Ltd. pp 92–3.

Thomas S (1994 e) Iodosorb ointment. In Thomas S, (Ed) Handbook of Wound Dressings (1994 Edition) London: Macmillan Ltd. pp 96–7.

Turner S (1985) Which dressing and why? In Westaby S, (Ed) Wound Care. London: Heinemann. pp 58–69.

Further Reading

Burns Unit, City Hospital, Nottingham (1995) Can you tell me why? A parents guide to treatment of a burn injury in their child. Nottingham: University of Nottinghan Printing and Photographic Unit.

Harding KG, Hughes LE, Markes J (1986) A Guide to the Practical Management of Granulating Wounds. Crewe: The Welcome Foundation.

Hooper W (1989) Life after a Burn. How to Cope at Home. Swindon: Jobst Zimmer Surgical Specialities, UK.

Kemble JVH, Lamb BE (1987) Practical Burns Management. London: Hodder and Stoughton.

Lawrence C (1992) Antibacterial prophylaxis in burns and other surface wounds. Wound Management 2 (2): 13–15.

Mason S, Forshaw A ( ) Burns Aftercare. A Booklet for Parents. Pan Med Limited.

Mason S, Turner H, Foley A ( ) Burns Aftercare. A Booklet for Patients at Home after Injury. Essex, UK: Smith and Nephew Pharmaceuticals.

Morgan B, Wright M (1986) Essentials of Plastic and Reconstructive Surgery. London: Faber and Faber.

Spencer KE (1990) A logical approach. Professional Nurse. 5 (6): 303–7.

Chapter 25
Care of a patient with a split skin graft donor site

A donor site is an area of the body used to provide a split skin graft (Coull, 1991 a) to resurface a burn wound (Konop, 1991). Several areas of the body can be used as a donor site including, chest, back, scalp and arms but more commonly the thighs and buttocks are used (Coull, 1991 a,b).

The selection of the donor site depends on the availability of skin and, in patients with extensive burns, it may not be possible to select preferred donor sites. It is then a case of using whatever skin is available.

Donor skin can be harvested using a variety of instruments, e.g. electric dermatome (Coull, 1991 a), air driven dermatome or a Watson knife. However, regardless of the method used the removal of a split thickness skin graft essentially results in a partial thickness wound. Both methods leave the deeper elements of the epidermis and dermis *in situ* which will regenerate the epidermal cells to allow the donor site to heal (Coull, 1991 b).

Some modern dressing materials have been used successfully to treat donor sites and these include semi-permeable films, hydrocolloid materials and alginates (Lawrence, 1989). A calcium/sodium alginate dressing is recommended as a primary dressing for split skin graft donor sites due to its haemostatic properties (Attwood, 1989; Vanstraelen, 1992; Thomas, 1994).

Regardless of the method of treatment the donor site will usually heal in about 7–10 days and can then be used to harvest more donor skin. However, subsequent skin grafts will be thinner and of poorer quality.

It is important to explain to the patient that postoperatively the donor site will be more painful than the graft site but this will gradually subside (Alderman, 1988). As healing occurs, the donor site may become itchy and the patient should be advised not to scratch. Antihistamines are usually prescribed by the medical staff and should be administered according to the patient's prescription chart as required.

1. Procedure for the preoperative care of a split skin graft donor site

In order to minimise the risk of wound infection the donor site needs to be as free from micro-organisms as possible.

To ease the shaving of split skin from a donor site the skin needs to be smooth and hair free. Any hairs transferred from the donor site to the recipient site may cause small pockets of infection and prevent the adherence of the skin graft thus lengthening the healing time. The procedure is usually performed in the Burns Unit operating theatre immediately prior to surgery. The patient may already be anaesthetised.

See sections 1, 2 and 4 (if applicable) for advice on procedures and sharps policy.

Equipment

Trolley/tray
Disposable razor
Sharps box
Soap
Water
Towel
Patient's own electric razor (optional)
Depilatory cream (optional)

Action	Rationale
Pre-operatively discuss with the medical staff and the patient the preferred donor site.	To ensure preparation of the correct donor site.
Immediately prior to surgery, in the operating theatre, prepare the proposed donor site.	In the hours before theatre, any abrasions and cuts sustained during shaving may become rapidly colonised with micro-organisms (Winfield, 1986; Llewellyn-Thomas, 1990).
On doctor's instructions: Using soap, water and a new razor blade, or the patient's own electric razor, shave the selected site and dry with the towel.	To minimise this risk shaving should take place immediately prior to surgery and not before. Wet shaving is less traumatic to the skin than dry shaving. There is less risk of abrasions and cuts using an electric razor (Petterson, 1986).
If the patient has requested the use a depilatory cream, follow the manufacturer's guidelines and use a test patch the night before surgery.	To ascertain if the patient is allergic to the cream.
If no reaction occurs, remove hair from the selected site using the depilatory cream.	The use of depilatory cream to remove hair has been shown to be associated with a lower post-operative infection rate and is also more cost effective (Seropian and Reynolds, 1991; Winfield, 1986).
Record in the appropriate nursing documentation and on the preoperative theatre documentation.	To maintain an accurate record.

2. Procedure for the postoperative care of a split skin graft donor site

See sections 1–5 in Chapter 1 for advice on procedures.

Equipment

Trolley
Sterile dressing pack
Sterile scissors
1 pair of unsterile gloves
1 pair of sterile gloves
Normal saline and alcohol swab
Alginate/hydrocolloid dressing of choice
Sterile gauze
Gamgee
Crepe bandage (of appropriate size)
Adhesive tape
Bacteriological wound swab (optional)
Moisturising cream (of choice)
Disposal bag
Patient's prescription chart

Action	Rationale
Administer analgesia as required and position the patient comfortably.	To minimise pain and discomfort for the patient. The donor site, by its nature, has many superficial nerve endings exposed and is, therefore, extremely painful (Coull, 1991 a).
Apply unsterile gloves when caring for the donor site (especially if it is leaking).	For the protection of the nurse against body fluids.
Postoperatively check the donor site 4 hourly.	To detect signs of excess oozing and/or haemorrhage (Coull, 1991 a).
If the dressing becomes wet, remove the outer bandage and any wet dressings underneath as far as the alginate dressing if necessary.	To minimise the risk of infection and for the comfort of the patient. Wet dressings lose their bacterial barrier properties in the presence of moisture (Lawrence, 1989).
	Calcium alginate dressings on split skin graft donor sites has been shown to give a highly significant improvement on healing and patient comfort (Attwood, 1989) and is recognised as a donor site haemostat (Groves and Lawrence, 1986).

Action	Rationale
Do not remove any dressings that are adherent.	Pulling at adherent dressings may destroy the ingrowth of capillaries.
Discard the dressings into the disposal bag, remove gloves and wash hands.	To minimise the risk of cross infection.
Apply sterile gloves and redress the site (on top of the alginate dressing) with sterile gauze, Gamgee and crepe bandage. Secure with adhesive tape.	To absorb any further wound exudate. Tape is preferable to pins for the safety of the patient.
Continue to repeat the above three actions whenever the dressing becomes wet or contaminated, noting the type of oozing, e.g. blood or serous fluid and if there is any noticeable odour. Report to the nurse in charge, as appropriate.	Continuous bleeding may indicate a bleeding point which may require surgical intervention or haemostatic dressings.
Offer the patient regular analgesia and monitor effectiveness.	Analgesia is recommended to encourage early mobilisation and minimise the risk of deep vein thrombosis (Coull, 1991 a).
If the dressing becomes green and/or offensive smelling apply unsterile gloves, remove the outer bandage and gauze layers as far as the alginate dressing.	To minimise the risk of infection. Pseudomonas aeruginosa produces a foul smelling bright green exudate and indicates infection is present in the donor site (Coull, 1991 a).
If any of the gauze is adherent, the area should be irrigated with normal saline.	Moistening the area will help to loosen the adherent areas. The use of antiseptics should be avoided as they increase the inflammatory response (Brennan and Leaper, 1985).
If the alginate dressing is adherent to the area, it should be irrigated with normal saline.	To facilitate easy removal and to avoid undue friction to the wound destroying new epithelial cells.
Discard into the disposal bag, remove gloves and wash hands.	To minimise the risk of cross infection.
If there is any discharge from the site a bacteriological wound swab should be taken for culture and sensitivity. Label and send to the microbiology laboratory.	Culture and sensitivity allows detection of infection which may cause deterioration of the wound.
Apply sterile gloves.	
If any exudate is present, irrigate the site with normal saline.	To remove excess exudate. Irrigation with warmed saline or water using a syringe may be sufficient to dislodge particles (Cutting, 1990; Stringer et al., 1983; Morison, 1992).

Action	Rationale
Assess the donor site for signs of infection and report any abnormalities to the nurse in charge.	Infection may cause deterioration of the wound and delay the healing process.
Redress the site:	To provide the optimum wound dressing and to encourage wound healing.
Apply Silver Sulphadiazine cream and cover with layers of paraffin gauze and Gamgee.	Silver Sulphadiazine cream and acetic acid are effective in treating pseudomonas infections (Coull, 1991 a).
Cover the wound with a single layer of paraffin gauze and apply gauze soaked in acetic acid solution and a padded layer of Gamgee. Secure with crepe bandage and adhesive tape.	Tape is preferable to pins for the safety of the patient.
Assess the donor site dressings daily and redress every 2–3 days or more often as the wound dictates.	For the comfort of the patient and to minimise the risk of cross infection.
If the dressing remains dry after 3–4 days, reduce the size of the dressing by removing some of the outer layers. **Do not** remove any adherent alginate.	For the comfort of the patient.
Apply one or two layers of sterile gauze and secure with crepe bandage and adhesive tape.	To absorb any further exudate. Tape is preferable to pins for the safety of the patient.
At 7 days postoperatively, soak off the alginate dressing in a bath or shower.	Moistening the area helps to loosen the adherent alginate dressing (Attwood, 1989).
If there are any unhealed areas redress using a selected alternative, e.g. hydrocolloid dressing.	To promote epithelialisation and maintain a moist environment for wound healing and to absorb any light wound exudate.
When the donor area is healed. Educate the patient on how to wash, moisturise and protect the area (see section 3 below).	For the comfort of the patient.
Record in the appropriate nursing documentation.	To maintain an accurate record.
Record the type of any wound care products used on the patient's prescription chart.	In accordance with unit policy/procedure for nurses prescribing wound care products.

3. Procedure for the aftercare of a split skin graft donor site

The aim of aftercare of donor sites is to minimise scar formation and to maintain the integrity of the skin. Once the donor site has healed the new epithelial cells are quite immature and do not produce sufficient sebum either to moisturise or protect the skin against the sun. The area must be massaged regularly with an efficient moisturising cream and effective sunscreens applied if the area is to be exposed (Coull, 1991 a). Aftercare may be carried out by any carer who has had instruction on what should be done and why, or may be carried out by the patient him or herself. It will also give the patient an opportunity to discuss with the carer his or her fears and anxieties about altered body image.

See sections 1 in Chapter 1 for advice on procedures.

Equipment

Trolley or patient's bedside table
1 pair of unsterile gloves
Bowl of warm water
Patient's flannel or disposable wipes
Mild unscented soap
Towel
Non-perfumed oil-based moisturising cream
Elasticated bandage measure
Elasticated bandage (of appropriate size)
Applicator
Patient's prescription chart

Action	Rationale
Ensure the patient is in a comfortable position.	For the comfort of the patient.
Wash hands and apply unsterile gloves.	For the protection of the nurse and to minimise the risk of cross infection.
Wash the healed donor site(s) with the non-perfumed soap and flannel or wipes.	A perfumed soap could irritate the skin. Soaping helps to prevent a build up of cream, which could lead to blocked pores.
Rinse the area(s) with clean water and pat dry with a towel, do not rub.	Rubbing dry can cause a breakdown of the skin, as the epithelium is still immature and delicate.
Massage the donor area(s) with the non-perfumed oil-based cream until it has been completely absorbed.	Massaging helps to break down the irregular formation of collagen fibres and promotes a good blood supply to the area.
	The new epithelial cells are immature and do not produce sufficient sebum to moisturise the

Action	Rationale
	skin. Moisturising cream should be applied regularly (Coull, 1991 a).
	Oil-based cream will prevent dryness caused by a lack of production of sebum.
Remove gloves and wash hands.	
Encourage the patient to participate in his or her own aftercare as much as possible.	To promote independence and encourage the patient to appreciate that this procedure will need to be carried out by him or her on discharge from hospital.
If applicable measure the donor area(s)/limb with the appropriate measure and choose the appropriate sized piece of elasticated bandage to cover the area.	To ensure the correct size for the patient.
Using the applicator, apply the elasticated bandage to the donor area, explaining to the patient the reason for its use and discuss future protection of the area(s).	Mechanical pressure is advised initially to minimise scarring until the scar maturation process is completed. In donor areas there are only a few melanocytes and little sebum; the areas should be protected from direct sunlight to prevent blistering from sunburn or effective sunscreens applied (Coull, 1991 a).
Ensure the patient is left feeling comfortable and allow time for discussion about altered body image.	To provide a safe environment. Open communication will help the patient to come to terms with his or her new skin appearance.
Repeat the above aftercare procedures at least three times a day.	This will result in supple skin with minimal scarring and irritation.
If the patient complains of itching administer antihistamine preparations as prescribed and encourage the patient not to scratch the area.	Itching is a frustrating effect of scarring (Cooper and Fenton 1996)
	Antihistamine preparations relieve itching and maintain the comfort of the patient. Scratching will cause damage to the new epithelial cells.
If the environment is warm try to keep the area cool and advise the patient to wear cotton clothes.	To relieve itching and for the comfort of the patient.

References

Alderman C (1988) Reconstructive approach. Nursing Standard 7 May: 24–5.

Attwood AI (1989) Calcium alginate dressing accelerates split skin graft donor site healing. British Journal of Plastic Surgery 43 (4): 373–9.

Brennan SS, Leaper DJ (1985) The effects of antiseptics on the healing wound. British Journal of Surgery 72: 708–82.

Cooper R, Fenton O (1996) Disfigurement and disablement In: Settle JAD Burns Management. Edinburgh: Churchill Livingstone.

Coull A (1991 a) Making sense of split skin grafts. Nursing Times 87 (40): 52–3.

Coull A (1991 b) Making sense of split skin grafts. Nursing Times 87 (27): 54–5.

Cutting K (1990) Wound cleansing. Surgical Nurse 3 (3): 4–8.

Groves AR, Lawrence JC (1986) Alginate dressing as a donor site haemostat. Annals of the Royal College of Surgeons of England 68: 27.

Konop D (1991) General local treatment. In Trofino RB Nursing Care of the Burn Injured Patient. Philadelphia: FA Davis Company. pp 62–3.

Lawrence JC (1989) Management of burns. The Dressing Times 2 (3): 1–4.

Llewellyn-Thomas A (1990) Pre-operative skin preparation. Surgical Nurse 3 (2): 24–6.

Morison M (1992) A colour guide to the nursing management of wounds. London: Wolfe.

Petterson E (1986) A cut above the rest. Nursing Times 82: 68–79.

Seropian R, Reynolds BM (1979) Wound infections after pre-operative depilatory versus razor preparation. American Journal of Surgery 121: 251–4.

Stringer M et al. (1983) Antiseptics and the casualty wound. Journal of Hospital Infection 4: 410–13.

Thomas S (1994) Kaltostat. In Thomas S, (Ed) Handbook of Wound Dressings (1994 Edition) London: MacMillan. pp 108–9.

Vanstraelen P (1992) Comparison of calcium sodium alginate (Kaltostat) and porcine xenograft (E–Z derm) in the healing of split thickness skin graft donor sites. Burns 18 (2): 145–8.

Winfield U (1986) Too close a shave. Nursing Times 82 (10): 64–8.

Further Reading

Burns Unit, City Hospital Nottingham (1995) Can you tell me why? A parent's guide to the treatment of a burn injury in their child. Nottingham: University of Nottingham Printing and Photographic Unit.

Hooper W (1989) Life After a Burn. How to Cope at Home. Swindon: Jobst Zimmer, Surgical Specialities Ltd., UK.

Kemble JVH, Lamb BE (1987) Practical Burns Management. London: Hodder and Stoughton.

Mason S, Forshaw A ( ) Burns Aftercare. A Booklet for Parents. Pan Med Limited.

Mason S, Turner H, Foley A ( ) Burns Aftercare. A Booklet for Patients at Home after Injury. Essex, UK: Smith and Nephew Pharmaceuticals.

Morgan B, Wright M (1986) Essentials of Plastic and Reconstructive Surgery. London: Faber and Faber.

Porter M (1992) Making sense of dressings. Wound Management 2 (2): 10–12.

Spencer KE (1990) A logical approach — Management of surgical wounds. Professional Nurse. 5 (6): 303–7.

Wilson GR, Taylor HE (1987) Blueprint for the Nursing Care of the Skin Graft Donor Site. Houndslow, Middlesex: Squibb Surgicare Limited.

Chapter 26
Care of a patient with a Wolfe graft

Wolfe grafts tend to give a much better result than split skin grafts, but because the donor site will need some form of repair they are only used for small to moderate areas.

Wolfe grafts are used frequently for secondary surgery to burns patients. They do not contract as much as split skin grafts so are useful for covering joints, as well as other areas such as eyelids and the corners of the mouth.

The care of these grafts is the same as for a split skin graft; however, when they are positioned in theatre, they are trimmed to fit the defect exactly. Because the graft is full thickness, it is more difficult for it to survive therefore it is used more widely on vascular areas.

For grafts to the face, the donor site is usually the postauricular area as this provides an ideal colour match (Grabb and Smith, 1979). For other areas, when larger grafts may be required, the groin is used.

The donor area is usually repaired by sutures, but occasionally, if a large area is involved, a split skin graft is used to repair the defect. The suture line or split skin graft donor area will require the care outlined in the appropriate procedures.

1. Procedure for care of a patient with a tie-over stitch pack following a Wolfe graft

A tie-over stitch pack secures and applies pressure to a skin graft. It is used where a traditional dressing might slip and/or where the patient might disturb the dressings. It is commonly used for grafts on the face and scalp, and also when the area to be grafted is in a cavity, e.g. following release of a contracture when pressure is needed to prevent haematoma formation between the bed and the graft (Macallan and Jackson, 1971). A split skin graft or a full thickness graft (Wolfe graft) may be used.

The tie-over pack consists of a layer of paraffin gauze (next to the graft) with a foam or wool pack on the top. When the graft is applied it overlaps the surrounding skin and when it is sutured in place the sutures go through the surrounding tissue, the graft and the dressing pack. The sutures are tied in the usual way but one end is left long. Once the areas surrounding the graft have been sutured, the long ends are tied together in the centre of the pack. This puts pressure on the graft and helps to prevent it from becoming detached from its bed (see Figure 26.1).

Graft sutured into defect
Sutures with one end left long

Foam or wool pack is laid over the layer of
paraffin gauze

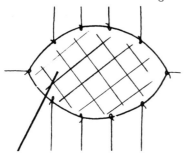

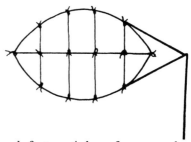

Layer of paraffin gauze applied over full thickness graft

Long end of sutures tied over foam or wool pack to hold it in place

Figure 26.1 *A tie-over pack.*

See sections 1–5 in Chapter 1 for advice on procedures.

Action	Rationale
Postoperatively elevate the limb on pillows or in a sling or sit the patient upright, well supported by pillows if the graft is on the face or scalp.	Elevation will help to reduce oedema and gravitational stasis.
Ensure that any pressure dressings are firmly applied.	The application of pressure will help to prevent fluid from collecting beneath the graft (Macallan and Jackson, 1971).
Discourage the patient from pulling at the dressing and check it regularly.	Any movement could prevent and/or damage the ingrowth of capillaries.
Commence 4 hourly observations of temperature and pulse. Report any abnormalities to the nurse in charge.	For early detection of infection.
The area around the graft should be inspected daily for cellulitis, pain or discharge.	For early detection of infection (Kemble and Lamb, 1984).
The area around the pack should be kept dry.	Uncontrolled moisture encourages the growth of micro-organisms.
Any discharge or oozing should be removed using an aseptic technique and normal saline.	To minimise the risk of cross infection.
	The use of antiseptics should be avoided as they can increase the inflammatory response (Brennan and Leaper, 1985).
The area should then be dried with gauze.	Gauze is preferable to cotton wool as there is less likelihood of the filaments of fibre adhering to the wound edges (Johnson, 1988).
(i) The graft is sutured into the defect. A full thickness graft is laid over	

Action	Rationale
If the discharge smells or is purulent then a bacteriological wound swab should be taken for culture and sensitivity, labeled and send to the microbiological laboratory.	Culture and sensitivity allows for suitable treatment to be instigated if there is deterioration of the wound.
Inform the nurse in charge and medical staff if infection is present. Subsequently:	Infection may warrant early removal of the pack.
Remove the pack and clean the graft using an aseptic technique.	To allow full assessment of the graft and minimise the risk of cross infection.
Treat the underlying infection.	To limit the damage to the graft.
Record in the appropriate nursing documentation.	To maintain an accurate record.

2. Procedure for removal of a tie-over stitch pack following a Wolfe graft

See sections 1–5 in Chapter 1 for advice on procedures and sharps policy.

Equipment

Trolley
Sterile dressing pack
1 pair of unsterile gloves
Sterile scissors or stitch cutter
2 pairs of sterile gloves
Sachet of normal saline and alcohol swab
Topical wound agents/wound sterile dressing (of choice)
Sterile gauze swabs
Gamgee (optional)
Crepe bandage (size appropriate to site)
Adhesive tape
Sharps box
Sterile 20 ml syringe (optional)
Disposal bag
Patient's prescription chart

Action	Rationale
Administer analgesia as prescribed approximately 30 minutes prior to commencing the procedure and position the patient comfortably.	To minimise pain and discomfort for the patient.

Action	Rationale
Apply unsterile gloves and remove the outer dressings. Discard into the disposal bag.	To minimise the risk of cross infection.
Remove gloves and wash hands. Apply sterile gloves.	To minimise the risk of cross infection.
Using the sterile scissors or stitch cutter, cut the long suture in the centre of the pack.	To prevent tension on the sutures when they are removed.
Cut and remove each suture around the circumference of the pack.	To facilitate easy removal of the pack.
Dispose of stitch cutter (if used) in the sharps box.	To prevent injury and in accordance with unit sharps policy.
Gently slide a pair of forceps or a gloved finger horizontally between the pack and the paraffin gauze while applying slight counterpressure onto the graft.	To prevent the graft being pulled from its bed when the pack is removed. The forceps are kept horizontal to prevent the points causing any trauma to the graft.
With a second pair of forceps or the gloved hand gently lift off the pack while still exerting gentle counterpressure onto the graft, using forceps or a gloved finger.	To facilitate easy removal of the pack.
If the pack is adherent, the area should be irrigated with saline.	Pulling will lift the graft from its bed and cause damage to the site. Moistening will help to loosen the adherent areas (Morgan and Wright, 1986).
Using the forceps or gloved hand gently lift off the paraffin gauze while exerting gentle counterpressure onto the graft, using forceps or a gloved finger.	To facilitate easy removal of the paraffin gauze.
If the paraffin gauze is adherent the area should be irrigated with saline.	Pulling will lift the graft from its bed and cause damage to the site. Moistening will help to loosen the adherent areas (Morgan and Wright, 1986).
Discard the pack into the disposal bag. Remove gloves, wash hands and apply second pair of sterile gloves.	To minimise the risk of cross infection.
If any exudate is present, irrigate the graft using warmed normal saline and a syringe.	To remove any debris while preventing damage to the ingrowth of capillaries from friction caused by cleaning (Leaper and Simpson, 1986).
	Irrigation with warmed saline or water using a syringe may be sufficient to dislodge particles (Cutting, 1990; Stringer et al., 1983; Morison, 1989).

Action	Rationale
Assess the graft for any skin loss, haematoma formation, and/or signs of infection. Report any abnormalities to the nurse in charge.	Haematoma formation and infection may cause skin loss. Extensive skin loss may require further skin grafting procedures.
Redress the graft using appropriate topical agents and wound dressing of choice, cover with secondary dressing, e.g. gauze, Gamgee (if required) and secure with bandage and adhesive tape.	To provide the optimum wound dressing. Gauze/Gamgee will absorb fluid and prevent outer dressings becoming moist. Bandages secure the dressing in place and the tape reduces friction and shearing forces which will occur if the dressing/bandages are loose. Tape is preferable to pins for the safety of the patient.
Record in the appropriate nursing documentation.	To maintain an accurate record.
Record the wound care product of choice on the patient's prescription chart	In accordance with unit policy/procedure for nurses prescribing wound care products.

3. Procedure for the care of a Wolfe graft donor site

The Wolfe graft donor site is usually in the groin or the postauricular area of the ear. It is usually repaired by a continuous suture which is removed 14–21 days postoperatively according to the doctor's instructions.

See sections 1–3 in Chapter 1 for advice on procedures.

Equipment

Clean tray
Bacteriological wound swab
Sterile dressing (of choice)
Hypoallergenic tape (optional)

Action	Rationale
Postoperatively check the donor site every 4 hours.	To detect signs of haemorrhage or oozing.
If the groin is used as a donor site keep the legs flexed for 24–48 hours.	To alleviate undue strain on the suture line in the groin.
Initially inspect the area around the donor site daily for cellulitis, pain or discharge.	For early detection of infection.
Ensure the area around the donor site is kept dry.	Uncontrolled moisture encourages the growth of micro-organisms.

Action	Rationale
Monitor and record temperature and pulse 4 hourly.	A rise in temperature may indicate signs of infection.
If there is any discharge from the site a bacteriological wound swab should be taken for culture and sensitivity, labelled and sent to the microbiology laboratory.	Culture and sensitivity allow detection of infection which may cause deterioration of the wound.
Cover the site with the sterile dressing of choice and secure with hypoallergenic tape, if required.	For protection of the wound against friction and to absorb any excess wound exudate.
Record in the appropriate documentation. If any abnormalities occur report to the nurse in charge.	To maintain an accurate record.
Record the dressing of choice on the patient's prescription chart.	In accordance with unit policy/procedure for nurses prescribing wound care products.

4. Procedure for the removal of a suture from a wolfe graft donor site

The suture from a Wolfe graft donor site is removed between 14 and 21 days postoperatively according to the doctor's instructions. It may be a continuous or subcuticular suture (see Figure 26.2).

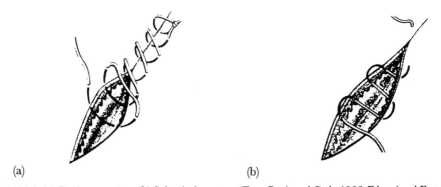

(a)   (b)

Figure 26.2 *(a) Continuous suture. (b) Subcuticular suture. (From Davis and Geck, 1992 Educational Factsheet; Suturing Techniques.)*

See sections 1, 2, 4 and 5 in Chapter 1 for advice on procedures and sharps policy.

Equipment

Trolley/tray
Sterile dressing pack
Sterile forceps/Spencer Wells forceps (optional)

1 pair of unsterile gloves
Sterile stitch scissors or stitch cutter
Sharps box
Disposal bag
1 pair of sterile gloves (optional)
Sachet normal saline and alcohol swab (optional)
20 ml sterile syringe (optional)
Sterile wound dressing (of choice)
Hypoallergenic tape (optional)
Patient's prescription chart

Action	Rationale
Assist the patient into a comfortable position which allows easy access to the donor site (suture line).	To facilitate the procedure for both the patient and the nurse.
If the donor site is covered put on the unsterile gloves and remove the dressing.	To minimise the risk of cross infection.
Discard the dressing into the disposal bag, remove gloves and wash hands.	To minimise the risk of cross infection.
Continuous suture:	The continuous suture technique involves making more than one stitch with a single strand of suture material before tying (Davis and Geck, 1992). A continuous suture line is as long as a line of interrupted sutures and has equal tension along its length.
– Using the forceps hold the knot on the top of the suture (at the end of the suture line). Gently lift upwards and cut the suture with the scissors or stitch cutter as close to the skin as possible and, exerting pressure gently but firmly, pull the suture out.	To minimise infection caused by drawing the exposed suture material through the subcutaneous tissue. To prevent undue pulling at the wound edges and to minimise pain.
– Repeat at each loop and continue down the wound until all the suture material has been removed.	To prevent future wound irritation or breakdown from suture material left in skin.
Subcuticular suture:	
– Cut the suture at one end of the wound leaving about 2.5 cm showing above the skin. Using forceps, or Spencer Wells forceps, grasp the long end of the suture at the other end of the wound and gently but firmly apply continuous traction in the long axis of the wound and pull the suture material out in one piece.	A subcuticular suture is another type of continuous suture. It is anchored at one end of the wound with a knot, then small stitches are made alternately on each side of the wound along the entire length. The suture is then pulled tightly to bring the wound edges together and tied.

Action	Rationale
Discard the suture material into the disposal bag.	To remove the suture material. To minimise the risk of cross infection.
If any exudate is present, apply sterile gloves and irrigate the wound with warmed normal saline.	To remove excess exudate (Cutting, 1990). Warmed fluids help to prevent a delay in wound healing (Lock 1980, Turner 1985). Saline is preferable to antiseptics (Brennan, Foster and Leaper 1986)
Assess the wound and cover (if required) with the sterile dressing (of choice) and secure with hypoallergenic tape (if required).	To absorb excess exudate. To provide the optimum wound dressing.
Dispose of the stitch cutter (if used) into the sharps box.	To prevent injury and in accordance with the local sharps policy.
Record the removal of the suture in the appropriate documentation.	To maintain an accurate record.
Record the wound dressing of choice on the patient's prescription chart.	In accordance with unit policy/procedure for nurses prescribing wound care products.

References

Brennan SS, Leaper DJ (1985) The effects of antiseptics on the healing wound. British Journal of Surgery 72: 780–2.

Brennan SS, Foster ME, Leaper DJ (1986) Antiseptic toxicity in wounds healing by secondary intention. Journal of Hospital Infection 8: 263–7.

Cutting KF (1990) Wound cleansing. Surgical Nurse 3 (3): 4–8.

Davis and Geck (1992) Suturing techniques — Educational fact sheet 10. Surgical Nurse 5 (1): 20–1.

Grabb WC, Smith JW (1979) Plastic Surgery (3rd Edition) Boston, MA: Little Brown.

Johnson A (1988) The cleansing ethic. Community Outlook February: 9–10.

Kemble JC, Lamb BE (1984) Plastic Surgery and Burns Nursing. London: Baillière Tindall.

Leaper DJ, Simpson RA (1986) The effects of antiseptics and antimicrobials on wound healing. Journal of Antimicrobial Chemotherapy 17 (12): 125–37.

Lock P (1980) Proceedings of the Symposium on Wound Healing. Gothenburg: Linden and Sonner.

Macallan ES, Jackson IT (1971) Plastic Surgery and Burns Treatment. London: Heinemann.

Morgan B, Wright M (1986) Essentials of Plastic and Reconstructive Surgery. London: Faber and Faber.

Morison M (1989) Wound cleansing — Which solution. Professional Nurse. February issue 220–5.

Morison M (1992) A Colour Guide to the Nursing Management of Wounds. London: Wolfe Publishing.

Stringer M et al. (1983) Antiseptics and the casualty wound. Journal of Hospital Infection 4: 410–13.

Turner S (1985) Which dressing and why? In Westaby S (Ed) Wound Care. London: Heinemann. pp 58–69.

Chapter 27
Care of a patient with a flap

A flap is a section of epidermis, dermis and subcutaneous tissue which can be combined with muscle and bone and moved from one part of the body to another (Kemble and Lamb, 1984) providing a vascular pedicle is maintained between the flap and the body for nourishment.

With advances in microsurgery free flaps can be used where an artery and a vein can be detached from their normal blood supply (at the pedicle) and the vein and artery anastomosed to an undamaged artery and vein adjacent to the skin loss. It may be used on the leg or scalp.

Types of flaps (Morgan and Wright, 1986)

The different types of flap are shown in Figures 27.1–6.

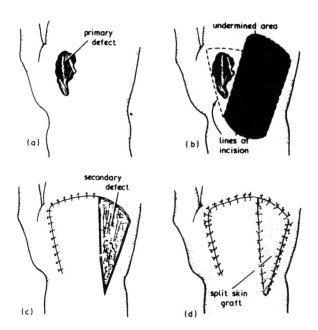

Figure 27.1 *A transposition flap.*

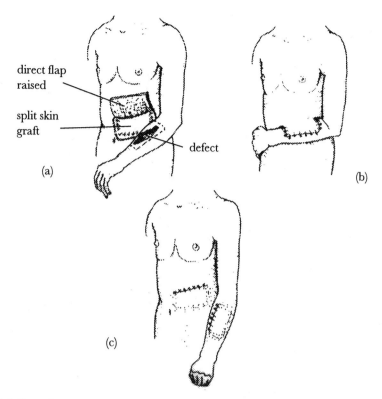

Figure 27.2 *A distant flap.*

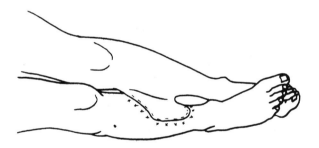

Figure 27.3 *A cross leg flap.*

Indications for use

1. When muscle and/or bone is required to cover a defect.
2. When subcutaneous tissue and skin must be transferred such as when a large defect requires covering.
3. To cover bare bone, tendon, cartilage and nerves (on which a skin graft would not take).
4. In poorly nourished people and those with a poor vascularity: flaps take more readily than grafts as they have their own blood supply.

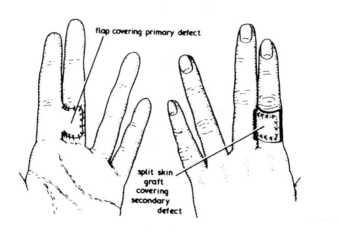

Figure 27.4 *A cross finger flap.*

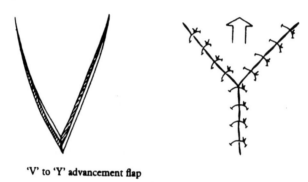

Figure 27.5 *A "V" to "Y" advancement flap.*

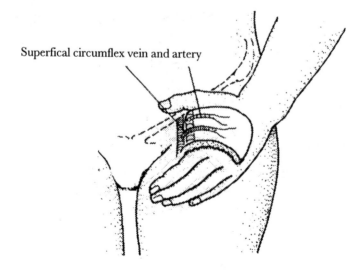

Figure 27.6 *A groin flap.*
(Figures 27.1–27.6 are taken from Morgan B, Wright M (1986) Essentials of Plastic and Reconstructive Surgery. Faber and Faber, reproduced with permission.)

Factors causing flap death (Kemble and Lamb, 1987)

A flap may fail because of either extrinsic or intrinsic factors. Kerrigan (1983) considers the only known intrinsic factor is inadequate nutrient bloodflow. Without an arterial blood flow, tissues will not survive.

Extrinsic causes of flap failure may be systemic or local.

1. Tension. Stretching a flap narrows and eventually obliterates the smaller blood vessels. This is recognised as a white area on the flap. Repositioning the two ends of the flap closer together may restore the circulation provided this is done before thrombosis occurs.
2. Infection. Beta haemolytic streptococci group A infection releases toxins which attack healing tissue and can cause accumulation of pus under a flap which may prevent adherence (Coull and Wylie, 1990).
3. Smoking increases the risk of platelet aggregation resulting in blood clots in the vascular system. A lowered haemoglobin decreases the oxygen-carrying capacity of the blood and reduces the amount of nutrients reaching the flap (Coull and Wylie, 1990).
4. Nutrition. Mahon (1987) considers nutritional status to be very important. A reduced level of plasma proteins will reduce osmotic pressure resulting in accumulation of fluid in the tissue spaces, non-adherence of the flap and may lead to flap necrosis (Coull and Wylie, 1990). A positive nitrogen balance promotes wound healing and a negative balance may reduce blood supply to subcutaneous tissues and affect wound healing. A satisfactory potassium level is needed to meet requirements for tissue synthesis.
5. Kinking has the same effect as tension.
6. Haematoma formation. If this occurs beneath the flap it may distend it sufficiently to compromise its blood supply and act as a nucleus for infection.
7. Pressure. The flap should be left exposed to check the blood supply is not occluded by pressure (Coull and Wylie, 1990).
8. Gravity. Venous supply may be inadequate so the flap becomes congested and blue.
9. Arteriosclerosis. Patients with arteriosclerosis are more prone to necrosis, it is therefore best to avoid flaps in the elderly.

How to improve the circulation in a flap

1. Reposition the flap horizontally.
2. Evacuate haematomas.
3. Cooling may reduce metabolic needs.
4. Administration of intravenous dextran may increase capillary flow and reduce viscosity.

1. Procedure for the postoperative care of a flap

See sections 1–5 in Chapter 1 for advice on procedures and sharps policy.

Equipment

Trolley
Sterile dressing pack
1 pair of sterile gloves
Sachet of normal saline and alcohol swab
Sterile scissors/stitch cutter
Sterile gauze
Gamgee
1 pair of unsterile gloves
Flap observations chart
Temperature recording box
Skin temperature probes (optional)
Sharps box
Patient's prescription chart

Action	Rationale
Postoperatively, warm the environment to at least 20°C.	If the patient is cool, peripheral circulation is reduced increasing the blood viscosity and the risk of clotting (Coull and Wylie, 1990) and the blood supply to the flap may be impaired (Souter and McGregor, 1986).
Elevate the limb on pillows or in a sling or position the patient comfortably, well supported by pillows ensuring the flap is not kinked or under pressure.	Elevation will help to reduce oedema and establish gravitational stasis. The position of the flap will assist in maintaining viability.
Monitor and record the patient's blood pressure half to 1 hourly.	Abnormalities in blood pressure may cause complications within the flap. Hypotension may reduce arterial flow depriving the flap of nutrients. Hypertension may increase arterial flow causing congestion of the flap, increased risk of embolism and tissue infarction (Coull and Wylie, 1990).
Administer regular analgesia as prescribed by the medical staff on the patient's prescription chart.	To minimise pain and discomfort of the patient. Patients undergoing stress or who are in pain release increased levels of glucocortisol which can affect tissues undergoing repair (Coull and Wylie, 1990).
Commence half to 1 hourly observations of the flap (or as directed by the medical staff) for 36 hours postoperatively.	Arterial occlusion can still occur up to 36 hours postoperatively (Souter and McGregor, 1986).

Action	Rationale
Record and report immediately any changes in the flap to the nurse in charge or medical staff.	Prompt action may improve the circulation of the flap.
Wherever possible, handle the flap as little as possible but if this is unavoidable strict hand-washing, the wearing of sterile gloves and a strict aseptic technique is essential.	To minimise the risk of infection.
Observe the colour of the flap and record on the appropriate chart.	The flap should be the same colour as the surrounding skin. A blue flap may indicate venous congestion, red may indicate infection, and white may indicate a poor arterial supply (Coull and Wylie, 1990).
Observe the temperature of the flap by placing the dorsum of one finger on the flap and comparing it to the surrounding skin.	The flap should feel the same temperature as the surrounding skin.
Place the skin probes onto the flap and surrounding skin (if requested by medical staff) monitor and record temperature measurements accordingly.	Skin temperature should be 34–36° C. A 2° C difference may indicate degeneration (Black and Black, 1987). If the flap feels warmer than the surrounding skin it may indicate an inflammatory response, e.g. infection.
	If the flap feels cooler, it may indicate poor arterial supply (Coull and Wylie, 1990).
If the flap is cool:	
— Cover with warm Gamgee.	Warming the flap will increase the blood supply.
— Check there is no pressure on the flap	Reducing pressure will avoid occlusion of the blood supply (Coull and Wylie, 1990).
If the flap is hot:	
— Inform the nurse in charge and the medical staff.	May indicate infection which could lead to degeneration of the flap.
Apply gentle finger pressure to the flap, release it and note the response time for the area to revascularise.	Capillary networks should ideally refill in 3 seconds, a delayed or absent refill may be due to arterial problems and an engorged flap may not blanche under pressure (Bonavita, 1985).
Feel the texture of the flap by applying gentle pressure with one finger and record.	If the flap feels hard, this may indicate haematoma formation, if spongy this may indicate arterial occlusion or kinking (Rodzwic and Donnard, 1986).

Action	Rationale
Observe and record any oozing or discharge: – Note the type and amount of fluid.	Pus may indicate infection, blood may indicate haematoma formation or an untied blood vessel.
– If the discharge smells or is purulent, take a bacteriological wound swab for culture and sensitivity, label and send to the microbiology laboratory.	Culture and sensitivity allows for suitable treatment to be instigated.
– Irrigate the area with warmed saline or clean the area using saline-soaked gauze.	Irrigation is recommended to remove debris and dislodge particles (Cutting, 1990). Warmed fluids help to prevent delays in wound healing caused by a drop in wound temperature (Turner, 1985). The use of antiseptics should be avoided as they increase the inflammatory response (Brennan and Leaper, 1985). Gauze is preferable to cotton wool as there is less likelihood of filaments of fibre adhering to wound edges (Wood, 1976).
– The area around the flap should be kept dry.	Uncontrolled moisture encourages the growth of micro-organisms.
Elevate the site so that drainage is away from the flap.	To reduce venous congestion — if it does not improve medical staff may prescribe leeches (see Section 2 below).
Express any haematomas by gently rolling sterile gauze applicators soaked in saline from the middle of the flap outwards.	Haematoma formation under the flap may compromise the blood supply and act as a nucleus for infection.
N.B. If unable to express the haematoma a suture may need to be removed using sterile scissors or a stitch cutter.	To allow the haematoma to be expressed.
If debris or exudate is present, clean the suture line gently with gauze soaked in warm saline or irrigate with saline using a syringe.	To remove debris and to allow assessment of the suture line. Gauze is preferable to cotton wool as there is less likelihood of filaments of fibre adhering to wound edges (Wood, 1976). Warm saline prevents spasm of blood vessels.
Check patency of any drainage tubes *in situ*, avoiding pressure on the flap.	To promote drainage, reduce haematoma formation and maintain a good blood supply to the flap (Coull and Wylie, 1990).
Remove drain when drainage is minimal and at the request of the medical staff.	
When handing over the care of the patient to another nurse, check the flap observations once together.	Individual nurses differ slightly in interpreting observations. By checking together, an understanding and agreement is obtained.

Action	Rationale
Ensure all observations are recorded in the appropriate nursing documentation and on the appropriate flap observation charts.	To maintain an accurate record.
Remove sutures 14–21 days postoperatively at the request of the medical staff.	To make sure the suture line is healed before removing sutures.
If the flap requires division, it is usually performed 14–21 days postoperatively and the patient may require anaesthesia.	To release the flap from its vascular pedicle and allow freedom of movement of the site.
Redress the wound with the sterile dressing of choice, cover with a secondary dressing (if required) and secure with bandage and/or adhesive tape as appropriate.	To provide the optimum wound dressing. To promote healing and minimise infection. To secure the dressing in place. Tape is preferable to pins for the saftey of the patient.
Record the wound care product on the patient's prescription chart.	In accordance with the unit policy/procedure for nurses prescribing wound care products.

2. Procedure for applying leeches

Leeches are parasitic worms of the class *Hirudinea* of which over 650 varieties are known (Coull, 1993). Leech therapy has been proven to be very useful in the treatment of venous insufficiency, this being a possible complication in newly replanted or transplanted tissues. Venous insufficiency or congestion will slow the arterial flow and eventually a clot will form cutting off the blood supply resulting in necrosis of the tissue (Danton, 1987).

The leech is placed onto the affected area and its salivary glands secrete a local anaesthetic. It then injects an anticoagulant — hirudin into the area along with a vasodilator which inhibits blood clotting (O'Hara, 1988). The leech will then feed for up to 40 minutes, although the procedure must be closely observed as the leech may drop off before this time. Following removal of the leech, the site will continue to ooze for up to 24 hours due to the effects of the hirudin. Applied 2–4 times daily the leech can remove between 20 and 60 ml of blood on each occasion depending on its size (Danton, 1987).

One of the problems associated with the use of leeches is the difficulty in getting the leech to attach itself to the tissue. This may be a sign that the problem is caused by arterial occlusion and not venous congestion (O'Hara, 1988). In these circumstances leeches must not be used because an endosymbiotic bacterium called *Aeromonas hydrophila* is present in the leech's gut, and this infection has been known to occur in patients following leech application to tissues with impaired arterial circulation. It has also been observed that if the leech is not easy to attach and does not feed well, the chances of the tissue reviving are decreased.

Before use, the leech should be kept cool at around 15° C and not exposed to sunlight (Biopharm, 1992).

Signs of arterial and venous occlusion are shown in Table 27.1.

Table 27.1 Signs of arterial and venous occlusion

	Arterial occlusion	**Venous congestion**
Skin colour	Pale, mottled blue	Cyanotic, blue
Capillary refill	Sluggish (> 2 sec)	Brisker than normal
Tissue turgor	Prune like, then hollow	Tense, swollen, distended
Temperature	Cool	Cool
Dermal bleeding	Serum and/or scant amount of dark blood	Rapid bleeding, dark blood

From O'Hara, 1988.

See sections 1–5 in Chapter 1 for advice on procedures.

Equipment

Trolley
Sterile dressing pack
Warm sterile water
Sachet of normal saline and alcohol swab
Sterile linen towel
1 pair of sterile gloves
Sterile gauze swabs
Leeches (available from pharmacy, must be prescribed)
Sugar solution (optional)
Alcohol wipe (optional)
Container with alcohol solution
Patient's prescription chart

Action	**Rationale**
Explain the need for leech therapy to the patient and answer any questions they may have, e.g. about pain.	The use of leeches can be repulsive to patients although many have been known to give their leech a name and dine out on the story for years (O'Hara, 1988). An anaesthetic substance released by the leech prevents the patient from feeling pain (Coull, 1993).
Explain to the patient that it is important not to touch the leech once it is in place.	So the leech does not become dislodged or attached to the patient's hand.
Apply sterile gloves.	To maintain asepsis.
Clean the flap or congested area with gauze soaked in warm water.	In order for the leech to attach itself adequately all contaminants must be removed, e.g. Povidone Iodine, old blood, etc. (Coull, 1993). Warmed fluids avoid a drop in wound surface temperature (Turner 1985)
Cover the surrounding area with a sterile linen towel. (If possible use a linen towel with a hole in it, or gauze soaked in water.)	To prevent the leech from migrating (Biopharm, 1992).

Action	Rationale
Using the forceps gently place the leech onto the site. **Do not** pick up the leech with your fingers.	Rough handling of the leech may injure its body. Using forceps prevents the leech from attaching itself to the nurse.
If the leech will not attach itself, apply a small amount of sugar solution to the desired area.	To encourage attachment of the leech (O'Hara, 1988).
Maintain close observation once the leech is in place.	To ensure that the leech has not migrated.
Check the area regularly. When the leech becomes engorged it will normally drop off independently. If not, remove by gently stroking it with an alcohol wipe. **Do not** pull the leech off.	Once the leech has taken its fill it releases a sucker and drops off leaving a triangular scar (Danton, 1987).
	Pulling the leech off the skin may cause the sucker to remain behind and cause a reaction or infection of the area (O'Hara, 1988; Coull, 1993).
	Using an alcohol wipe or sprinkling salt on the leech's head assists with removal (Cmiel, 1990).
Remove the leech and handle very gently.	In order to prevent regurgitation of the leech's gut contents which may cause *Aeromonas hydrophila* bacterium to spread into the wound (O'Hara, 1988).
N.B. Leeches are usually only used once and must only ever be used on the same patient. If the leech is to be used again, it can be made to regurgitate gut contents by leaving it in a 5% saline solution for 2–3 minutes.	Leeches do not feed very well a second time even following regurgitation. One leech must not be used on several patients due to transmission of infection, e.g. hepatitis B and HIV (Danton, 1987; Coull, 1993).
On completion, place the leech in a container with alcohol solution and send for incineration. Ensure the container is marked "used leeches".	To ensure a used leech is not used again by mistake.
When the leech has been removed, clean the area with warmed saline — the site may ooze for 4–6 hours and up to 24 hours after the leech has completed feeding.	Warmed fluids avoid a drop in wound surface temperature which may delay healing (Turner 1985)
	To minimise the risk of infection and to prevent clotting of the area. The leech can unclog the small veins by sucking out congested blood causing prolonged bleeding (Coull, 1993; Strangio, 1991).
Remove gloves and wash hands.	To minimise the risk of infection.

Action	Rationale
Ensure medical staff prescribe prophylactic antibiotics for the patient.	To minimise the risk of infection (Whitlock et al., 1983; Dickson, Bootham and Hare, 1984; Hermansdorfer et al., 1988).
Record in the appropriate documentation.	To ensure staff are aware of the type of treatment in use, and to evaluate if treatment was successful. To maintain an accurate record.
Apply further leeches on direction from the medical staff.	Until venous congestion appears to improve or if congestion returns when bleeding from the bite wound ceases (Coull, 1993).
Record the results of full blood counts in the nursing documentation.	Continued oozing from bite wounds may lead to a drop in haemoglobin (Coull, 1993).

3. Procedure for the care of a patient following a Z-plasty

A Z-plasty is performed in reconstructive burn surgery to release a contracture. It is a surgical procedure consisting of raising two triangular transposition flaps on either side of the contracted scar which is then removed. When the flaps are transposed, there is a lengthening effect and the scar tissue is transferred to a more advantageous position (See Figure 27.7).

See sections 1–5 in Chapter 1 for advice on procedures and sharps policy.

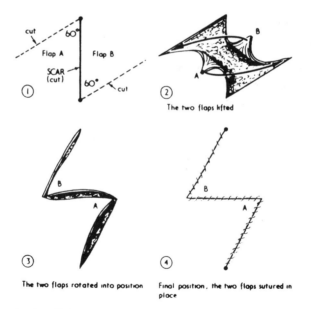

Figure 27.7 *The surgical procedure for a Z-plasty.*
(From Morgan B, Wright M (1986) Essentials of Plastic and Reconstructive Surgery. Faber and Faber, reproduced with permission.)

Equipment

Trolley
Sterile dressing pack
Sterile scissors/stitch cutter
1 pair of unsterile gloves
1 pair of sterile gloves
Sachet of normal saline and alcohol swab
Sterile gauze
Soft paraffin
Sterile towel
20 ml sterile syringe (optional)
Bacteriological wound swab
Sharps box
Disposal bag
Patient's prescription chart

Action	Rationale
Administer analgesia as prescribed and ensure the patient is in a comfortable position well supported by pillows.	To minimise pain and discomfort for the patient.
Elevate area/limb in a sling or support on pillows.	To reduce oedema and establish gravitational stasis.
Maintain a warm environment for the patient postoperatively of at least 20° C.	If the patient becomes cool, peripheral perfusion is reduced and the blood supply may be impaired.
Cover the area with a sterile towel.	To minimise the risk of cross infection.
Commence half to 1 hourly observations of the Z-plasty for at least 24 hours postoperatively.	To detect signs of impaired blood supply.
Record and report any changes in the Z-plasty immediately to the nurse in charge.	Prompt action may improve circulation to the Z-plasty.
Wherever possible avoid touching the suture line but if this is unavoidable, strict handwashing, the wearing of sterile gloves and a strict aseptic technique are essential.	To minimise the risk of infection.
Observe the colour of the flaps and record.	The flaps should be the same colour as the surrounding skin. Blue flaps may indicate venous congestion, red may indicate infection, and white may indicate a poor blood supply.

Action	Rationale
Observe the temperature of the flaps by placing the dorsum of one finger on each flap and compare it to the surrounding skin.	Aim for each flap to feel the same temperature as the surrounding skin. If the area around the Z-plasty feels hot, it may indicate infection which could lead to degeneration of the flap.
Feel the texture of the flaps by applying gentle pressure with one finger and record.	If any of the flaps feel hard this may indicate haematoma formation.
Express any haematomas from the suture line by gently rolling sterile gauze applicators soaked in saline from the outside of the Z-plasty inwards towards the sutures.	Haematoma formation may compromise the blood supply or cause tension on the suture line and act as a nucleus for infection.
N.B. If unable to express the haematoma using the sterile scissors or a stitch cutter remove 1–2 sutures.	To allow the haematoma to be expressed.
If debris or exudate is present clean the suture line gently with gauze soaked in saline or irrigate with saline using a syringe.	To remove debris and any dry blood and to allow assessment of the suture line. Gauze is preferable to cotton wool as there is less likelihood of filaments of fibre adhering to the wound edges (Wood, 1976).
Apply soft paraffin to the suture line.	To minimise the risk of crusty particles adhering to the suture line.
Cover the wound as appropriate or apply a non-adherent dressing if the patient is to be discharged from hospital.	To absorb excess exudate and for the comfort of the patient.
Record in the appropriate nursing documentation.	To maintain an accurate record.
If the patient is to be discharged from hospital advise them not to put too much strain on the suture line. However, they may return to work or school if no physical activity is involved.	To prevent rupturing of the suture line.
Remove sutures 14 days postoperatively unless otherwise instructed by the medical staff.	To allow the Z-plasty time to heal before the sutures are removed.

References

Biopharm UK (1992) Maintenance of Leeches. Hendy, Dyfed: Biopharm UK.

Black JM, Black SB (1987) Surgical management of pressure ulcers. Nursing Clinics of North America 22 (2): 429–38.

Bonavita L (1985) Knee tissue transfer. American Journal of Nursing 85: 384–7.

Brennan SS, Leaper D (1985) The effects of antiseptics of the healing wound. British Journal of Surgery 72: 780–2.

Cmiel P (1990) Post operative management of the replant. Patient monitoring, complications and education. Critical Care Nursing Quarterly 13 (1): 47–54.

Coull A, Wylie K (1990) Regular monitoring — The way to ensure flap healing. Professional Nurse October: 18–21.

Coull AF (1993) Using leeches for venous drainage after surgery. Journal of Wound Care 2 (5): 294–7.

Cutting K (1990) Wound cleansing. Surgical Nurse 3(3): 4–8.

Danton SS (1987) Fashionable blood suckers. Nursing Times 4 February: 53–4.

Dickson WA, Bootham P, Hare K (1984) An unusual source of hospital wound infection. British Medical Journal 289: 1727–8.

Hermansdorfer J, Lineaweaver W, Follansbee S, et al. (1988) Antibiotic sensitivities of aeromonas hydrophilia cultured from medical leeches. British Journal of Plastic Surgery 41: 649–51.

Kemble JH, Lamb BE (1984) Plastic Surgical and Burns Nursing. Eastbourne: Baillière Tindall.

Kemble JH, Lamb BE (1987) Practical Burns Management. London: Hodder and Stoughton.

Kerrigan CL (1983) Skin flap failure: pathophysiology. Plastic and Reconstructive Surgery 72(6): 766–74.

Mahon SM (1987) Nursing interventions for the patient with a myocutaneous flap. Cancer Nursing 10 (1): 21–31.

Morgan B, Wright M (1986) Essentials of Plastic and Reconstructive Surgery. London: Faber and Faber.

O'Hara MM (1988) Leeching: A modern use for an ancient remedy. American Journal of Nursing 88 (12): 1656–8.

Rodzwic D, Donnard J (1986) The use of myocutaneous flaps in reconstructive surgery for head and neck cancer. Guidelines for nursing care. Oncology Nursing Forum 3 (3): 29–34.

Souter DS, McGregor IA (1986) The radial forearm flap in oral reconstruction — The experience of sixty consecutive cases. Plastic and Reconstructive Surgery 78 (1): 1–18.

Strangio L (1991) Leeches when bleeding is exactly what you want RN 54 (9): 31–3.

Turner S (1985) Which dressing and why? In Westaby S (Ed) Wound Care. London: Heinemann. pp 58–69.

Whitlock MR, O'Hare PM, Sanders R, Morrow WC (1983) The medical leech and its use in plastic surgery. A possible cause for infection. British Journal of Plastic Surgery 36: 240–4.

Wood RAB (1976) Disintegration of cellulose dressings in open granulating wounds. British Medical Journal 785: 1444–5.

Further Reading

Baker CA, Nayduch DA (1989) Medicinal leech therapy: A case study. Orthopaedic Nursing 8 (2): 21–4.

Bates M, Kneer K, Logan C (1989) Medicinal leech therapy: An overview. Orthopaedic Nursing 8 (2): 12–17.

O'Hara MM (1991) Beauty and the beast: Nursing care of the patient undergoing leech therapy. Plastic Surgical Nursing 11 (3): 101–4.

Suster V, Giormuso C (1991) A policy and procedure for the use of leeches. Plastic Surgical Nursing 11 (3): 107–9.

Chapter 28
Care of a patient with a tissue expander

Tissue expanders are used to expand the size of a flap for reconstructive surgery and to reduce the size of the donor site (Reynolds, 1992). The tissue expander is a silicone bag or balloon which is inserted into a subcutaneous pocket and is slowly expanded by injecting sterile normal saline over a period of weeks/months via a gel-filled valve. This is connected to the tissue expander by a filling tube, which is inserted under the subcutaneous layer of the skin. Tissue expanders are most commonly round or rectangular in shape (Reynolds, 1992).

As the tissue expander is inflated, the internal pressure exerts force on the flap and causes the soft tissue to expand. When the expander is removed the expanded soft tissue is then ready to use as an advancement flap.

Advantages (Sharpe, 1987)

1. Tissue expansion utilises local tissue of good colour and texture match, and retains sensation and hair-bearing characteristics (Wyllie, Gowar and Levick, 1986).
2. Stretching local tissue results in fewer scars.
3. There is less donor site morbidity in scarring, and less contour defects.
4. Flexible expansion programme.
5. It is repeatable if it fails.
6. Pain and scarring of graft donor sites are avoided.

Disadvantages (Sharpe, 1987)

1. It is a slow process which cannot be achieved in one session.
2. Frequent inflation requires intensive manpower and frequent hospital visits.
3. It may be unsuitable in some areas where there is a danger of contractures developing.
4. Contour problems may occur due to a loss of subcutaneous fat.
5. The tissue expander becomes uncomfortable when it is fully inflated and the patient may be unable to bath unaided. Clothes may not fit and the patient may feel too self-conscious to go out. No physical exercise or rough play is allowed due to the danger of splitting both the tissue expander and the skin.

6. In a young child it is difficult to explain about the tissue expander and why it is being inflated (Martin, 1995).

Complications (Wyllie, Gowar and Levick, 1986)

1. Infection.
2. Haematoma formation.
3. Necrosis.
4. Ischaemia and wound breakdown.
5. Implant failure/rupture.
6. Pressure caused by inflated tissue expander.
7. Neurological problems.
8. Insufficient expansion.
9. Skin changes.
10. Bony indentations.
11. Late problems with scars.

1. Procedure for the postoperative care of a patient with a tissue expander

See sections 1–5 in Chapter 1 for advice on procedures.

Equipment

Trolley
1 pair of unsterile gloves
Appropriate observation charts
Sterile dressing (if required, as appropriate)
Sterile gloves
Sachet of normal saline and alcohol swab
Sterile dressing (of choice)
Sterile gauze
Adhesive tape
Patient's prescription chart

Action	Rationale
Position the patient on his or her side so that no pressure is on the tissue expander. When awake and alert assist the patient to sit up.	To help maintain airway by preventing tongue obstructing pharynx. To enable the lungs to expand to prevent chest infection.
Check oxygen and suction are working next to patient's bedside.	Oxygen may be prescribed postoperatively by the anaesthetist and may be required if the patient becomes cyanosed. Suction may be required if the patient has excessive oral secretions and is unable to swallow or "spit out". To maintain the airway.

Action	Rationale
Place vomit bowl and tissues next to the patient's bed.	For the patient's comfort especially if they feel nauseated postoperatively and vomit.
– Offer mouthwashes if the patient vomits. – Record and report any vomiting. – Administer antiemetics as prescribed by the medical staff.	For the patient's comfort. To maintain an accurate record. To prevent the patient vomiting, thereby maintaining the comfort of the patient.
Administer analgesia as prescribed by the medical staff.	To minimise pain and discomfort for the patient.
Administer antibiotics as prescribed by the medical staff.	To minimise the risk of infection.
Record pulse and respirations on return from the operating theatre then quarter hourly slowly reducing to half hourly, 2 hourly and 4 hourly when stable and within normal limits for the age of the patient. Report any significant changes to the nurse in charge.	Observe for an increasing pulse rate indicating pain, haemorrhage or anxiety. Analgesia may depress the respiratory rate, and irregular respiration rates may indicate haemorrhage.
If the patient has a diamorphine infusion in progress, record 1 hourly observations of the respiratory rate. **N.B. If the respiration rate falls below 12 breaths per minute, switch the infusion off and inform the nurse in charge.**	Diamorphine may depress the respiratory rate.
Observe if the patient becomes restless. Administer analgesia and/or oxygen as appropriate and report to nurse in charge.	May be caused by pain, anxiety, hypoxia.
Record the patient's temperature on return from the operating theatre, if within normal limits record 4 hourly.	
If pyrexial:	May indicate infection.
– Record hourly	
– Administer antipyretics as prescribed and report any abnormalities to nurse in charge.	There is a risk of febrile convulsion in young children with pyrexia.
If the patient is cold (with a temperature below 36.5° C)	
– Cover the patient with extra blankets. – Monitor temperature hourly until within normal limits.	The patient may become hypothermic following the anaesthetic.

Action	Rationale
Record when the patient has passed urine.	Anaesthetic can cause urine retention.
Observe the wound site for:	
– Bleeding.	Haemorrhage may indicate untied blood vessel.
– Oozing or discharge of pus.	Pus may indicate infection.
– Oedema.	
– Bruising at the wound site.	
– Record and report amount and type of above.	To maintain an accurate record.
Dress the expander site with a Povidone Iodine or an alternative antibacterial agent daily.	To minimise the risk of infection. Povidone Iodine is an ideal topical agent (Reynolds, 1992).
Check the wound site does not become red, inflamed or painful. Assess the suture line regularly if exposed and remove any exudate by irrigating with warmed saline.	For early detection of infection so that appropriate antibiotics can be prescribed. To minimise the risk of infection. Warmed fluids help to prevent delays in wound healing caused by a drop in wound temperature (Tumei, 1985). The use of anticeptics should be avoided as they increase the inflammatory response (Brennan and Leaper 1985)
Position the patient so that no pressure is put onto the tissue expander or entry port and the patient is comfortable.	To minimise the risk of pain and discomfort for the patient.
Check the patency of any wound drains *in situ*, empty and record type and amount of drainage daily. Remove as directed by medical staff when drainage is minimal.	To prevent formation of a haematoma. To maintain an accurate record.
Check i.v. cannula site does not become red or inflamed or painful and give i.v. fluids as prescribed. Discontinue at doctor's request. Commence clear fluids (as tolerated) when the patient is awake and alert.	To observe for signs of infection and to prevent dehydration. There is a risk of inhaling fluid until fully conscious. If the patient is started on a normal diet immediately there is an increased risk of vomiting.
Remove sutures at doctor's request (about 2 weeks postoperatively).	
On discharge, give follow up information and date for first inflation of tissue expander.	

2. Procedure for the inflation of a tissue expander

Inflation usually begins 1–2 weeks after insertion of the tissue expander and the procedure may be repeated once or twice a week depending on the patient's convenience
until adequate expansion has been achieved (this decision will be made by the medical
staff). This procedure is indicated as an expanded role for nurses on the Burns Unit.

See sections 1–5 in Chapter 1 for advice on procedures and sharps policy.

Equipment

Trolley
Sterile dressing pack
1 pair of sterile gloves
Sterile gauze
Tube of local anaesthetic cream (optional)
Sterile semi-permeable film dressing (optional)
Sterile needle (of appropriate size)
Sterile 60 ml syringe
Butterfly cannula
100 ml bottle of sterile normal saline and alcohol swab
Paper tissues
Small sterile adhesive plaster
Alcohol-based wipe
Sharps box

Action	Rationale
One hour prior to inflation apply local anaes-thetic cream to port site and cover with semi-permeable film dressing.	Local anaesthetic cream takes at least 1 hour to have an effect and minimises pain on insertion of the needle through the skin to the port site.
Prior to commencing the procedure remove the semi-permeable film dressing and wipe the local anaesthetic cream from the skin using tissues.	To allow access to the port site.
Observe the entry port site, filling tube site and tissue expander site for pain, redness and inflammation. Report any abnormalities to the nurse in charge.	To detect signs of infection. The presence of infection may indicate the tissue expander will need to be removed.
Palpate the site of tissue expander. The size should relate to the amount of fluid in situ. Report any abnormalities to the nurse in charge.	Inability to palpate the site when fluid has been inserted may indicate that the tissue expander is leaking.

Action	Rationale
Observe the colour of the skin over the tissue expander site. It should be the same colour as the surrounding skin. Report any abnormalities to the nurse in charge.	Redness may indicate infection. When the tissue expander has been inflated, the pressure may cause blanching of the skin, necrosis, tissue breakdown, or extrusion of the prosthesis (Cullen and Clarke, 1986).
Assist the patient into a comfortable position ensuring there is no pressure on the tissue expander site. Ask the patient to remain as still as possible.	For the comfort of the patient. Pressure on the site may restrict expansion. If the patient moves there is a risk of the needle missing the entry port.
Wash hands and apply sterile gloves.	To minimise the risk of cross infection.
Draw up the required volume of sterile saline into the syringe via the sterile needle.	To assist with early preparation of equipment for later use.
Clean the skin over the entry port site using an alcohol-based wipe and allow to dry.	To minimise the risk of cross infection.
Using a gloved hand, palpate the area over the entry port site and with the other hand insert the butterfly cannula through the skin into the entry port.	To identify the port and facilitate direct access of the butterfly cannula (Radovan, 1984; Reynolds, 1992).
Attach the syringe to the butterfly cannula.	A butterfly cannula is easier to connect and disconnect to a syringe than an injection needle.
Slowly inject the sterile normal saline 5 ml at a time (volume requested by medical staff) until: – The skin over the tissue expander becomes white. – The syringe springs back on itself.	The tissue expander is inflated to its maximum expansion on each occasion.
If the patient complains of discomfort or pain, or if the overlying skin blanches, slowly withdraw some of the saline into the syringe until normal skin colour returns.	Too much fluid may have been inserted into the tissue expander at one time. If the saline is not withdrawn and pressure released, necrosis may occur (Radovan, 1984). Patient feedback is an accurate guide to adequate expansion (Reynolds, 1992).
Check the patient feels comfortable before removing the syringe and butterfly cannula.	To minimise pain and discomfort after the procedure and to avoid the butterfly cannula having to be reinserted later.
Cover the entry port site with a small adhesive plaster.	To minimise the risk of cross infection (Reynolds, 1992).
Complete the appropriate nursing documentation, record the date and amount of fluid inserted into the tissue expander and any complications.	To maintain an accurate record of the total amount of fluid inserted into the tissue expander to date.

Action	Rationale
Palpate the site of the tissue expander. The size should relate to the amount of fluid *in situ*. Report any abnormalities to the nurse in charge.	To detect for signs of leakage.
Re-emphasise to the patient the importance of caring for the site, e.g. avoiding trauma and noting any signs of pain, redness and swelling.	To minimise the risk of rupturing the tissue expander and early detection of complications, e.g. infection.
Discuss with the patient the date for the next inflation as requested by the medical staff.	To maintain continuity of treatment and for the convenience of the patient.
Psychological support/counselling must be given continually throughout the procedure by medical and nursing staff (Reynolds, 1992).	Many patients find the procedure mentally and physically distressing (Reynolds, 1992).

References

Brennan SS, Foster ME, Leaper DJ (1986) Antiseptic toxicity in wounds healing by secondary infection. Journal of Hospital Infection. 8: 263–7.

Cullen KW, Clarke JA, McLean WR (1986) Complications of tissue expansion in the burned scalp. Burns 12: 273–6.

Lock P (1980) Proceedings of the Symposium on Wound Healing. Gothenburg: Linden and Sonner.

Martin V (195) A strategy for helping a child with burn injuries to cope with reconstructive surgery. Journal of Wound Care 4 (1): 46–8.

Radovan C (1984) Tissue expansion in soft tissue reconstruction. Plastic and Reconstructive Surgery October: 482.

Reynolds J (1992) Tissue expansion. British Journal of Nursing 1 (3): 134–6.

Sharpe DT (1987) Tissue expansion. Burns 13: 43–8.

Turner S (1985) Which dressings and why? In Westaby S (Ed) Wound Care. London: Heinemann. pp 58–69.

Wyllie FJ, Gower JP, Levick PL (1986) Use of tissue expanders after burns and other injuries. Burns 12: 277–82.

Further Reading

Brunner LS, Suddarth DS (1981) The Lippincott Manual of Paediatric Nursing. London: Harper and Row.

Lewer H, Robertson L (1987) Care of the Child. London: MacMillan Education.

Manders EK, Scherden MJ, Furry JA, et al. (1984) Soft tissue complications. Plastic and Reconstructive Surgery 74 (4): 493–507.